# 50 things you can do today to manage hay fever

### Wendy Green

Foreword by John Collard

Clinical Adviser, Allergy UK

## PERSONAL HEALTH GUIDES

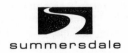

summersdale

50 THINGS YOU CAN DO TODAY TO MANAGE HAY FEVER

Summersdale Publishers Ltd
46 West Street
Chichester
West Sussex
PO19 1RP
UK

www.summersdale.com

Printed and bound in Great Britain

ISBN: 978-1-84953-017-0

Substantial discounts on bulk quantities of Summersdale books are available to corporations, professional associations and other organisations. For details contact Summersdale Publishers by telephone: +44 (0) 1243771107, fax: +44 (0) 1243 786300 or email: nicky@summersdale.com.

Disclaimer
Every effort has been made to ensure that the information in this book is accurate and current at the time of publication. The author and the publisher cannot accept responsibility for any misuse or misunderstanding of any information contained herein, or any loss, damage or injury, be it health, financial or otherwise, suffered by any individual or group acting upon or relying on information contained herein. None of the opinions or suggestions in this book is intended to replace medical opinion. If you have concerns about your health, please seek professional advice.

To my husband Gordon, thanks for being so
supportive

# Acknowledgements

I'd like to thank John Collard, Clinical Director at Allergy UK, for kindly agreeing to write a foreword. Thanks also to Jennifer Barclay for commissioning this book and to Anna Martin and Sarah Scott for their very helpful editorial input.

# Contents

9. Clear up pet hair/dander

10. Clean your home naturally

11. Make your home a smoke-free zone

12. Cut back on dairy products

13. Consider eating less wheat

14. Eat foods high in essential fatty acids

15. Eat antioxidant-rich fruit and vegetables

16. Choose low GI foods

17. Drink green tea

18. Have a spoonful of honey

19. Boost your beneficial bacteria

20. Eat foods containing quercetin

21. Go for garlic

22. Soothe symptoms with supplements

23. Consider nutritional therapists' advice

24. Keep a stress diary

25. Try not to worry

26. Change your attitude

27. Simplify your life

28. Assert yourself

29. Seek support

30. Sleep soundly

31. Laugh more

32. Do something purely for pleasure

33. Get the exercise habit

34. Consider ecotherapy

35. Practise muscle relaxation

36. Meditate

# Author's Note

I was 18 when I began suffering from hay fever. I remember only too well how unbearably sore, gritty, watery and swollen my eyes were and how utterly miserable I felt that summer. To make matters worse, my symptoms returned in the autumn, which puzzled me at the time, as I wasn't aware that grass pollen wasn't the only culprit – other types of pollen released later in the year were to blame.

The following summer, whilst I was completing a secretarial course at my local college, my symptoms were so severe that I struggled to complete a shorthand exam and fled from the classroom, sobbing. Happily, I did pass the exam, but my low mood prompted me to return to my GP's surgery. My doctor assured me that it was normal to feel miserable when suffering from hay fever. I took the antihistamines he prescribed and found they helped my symptoms, but they made me feel drowsy, so I decided to find a more natural treatment.

The following year I began drinking cider vinegar with honey in a glass of water every morning, after reading that it could help. I discovered that the taste wasn't too bad, once I'd got used to it! My symptoms gradually subsided and didn't return until very recently. I'd like to think that my natural remedy did the trick, but I suspect that my symptoms disappeared of their own accord – apparently they often do. Another possibility is that, over the years, my daily dose of vitamin C has helped. Ironically, this summer – whilst writing this book – and for the first time in years, I've experienced mild symptoms affecting my nose and sinuses; I'm now following some of the tips outlined in this book and have already noticed an improvement! I believe that, although a predisposition to hay fever is largely inherited, it is possible to reduce the frequency and severity of your symptoms through preventative strategies and dietary and lifestyle changes.

Wendy Green

# Foreword

**by John Collard,**
**Clinical Director, Allergy UK**

All too often, hay fever is dismissed as a trivial complaint and is not taken seriously. It is the most common allergy, with millions of sufferers in the UK alone, many of them children or young adults. Hay fever has a huge impact on quality of life at work, at school and at home, but friends and relatives of sufferers are often unsympathetic or just get fed up with their spring or summer being ruined by their companions' constant symptoms. Hay fever often goes hand in hand with other problems such as eye or ear symptoms and sinus congestion, and it increases the risk of asthma. Despite this, even healthcare professionals are often dismissive of hay fever and fail to ensure that it is properly managed. The majority of sufferers just try and manage their symptoms as best they can; yet with the right information and management, almost everyone can get their symptoms under control. Modern methods of desensitisation to pollens are extremely effective for those people who cannot get proper relief from medication and other measures.

This excellent, well-researched book brings together a wealth of information about hay fever. Causes, symptoms and treatment options are discussed, along with an array of tips about self-management, products and alternative treatments, as well as sources of further information, help and advice. Despite the complexity of the subject, this book is easy to read and clear about the evidence supporting the advice. If you have hay fever (or year-round nasal symptoms) this invaluable book is the only one you need.

# Introduction

Summer should be the time when we all enjoy the great outdoors, but for around one in five people in the UK, it is blighted by the misery of hay fever. Hay fever is thought to affect three times as many people now as it did during the 1970s. The condition is especially common among young people – according to the *British Medical Journal*, over one in three teenagers in the UK suffer from it. Experts blame a number of factors for this increase, including higher standards of hygiene in our homes, the over-prescribing of antibiotics, global warming, pollution, our diets and our increasingly stressful lifestyles.

This book explains what hay fever is and how genetic, environmental, dietary and psychological factors can play a part in its development. It offers practical advice and a holistic approach to help you deal with your symptoms. You'll discover easy ways to reduce your exposure to pollen and simple dietary and lifestyle changes that may help to prevent and treat attacks. You'll also find stress management strategies and DIY techniques from complementary therapies. At the end of the book you'll find details of helpful products, books and organisations.

### Famous hay fever sufferers

Famous hay fever sufferers include the actress Scarlett Johansson, who complained of suffering from hay fever whilst filming *Match Point* and described how, in one scene, which was filmed in a wheat field, one of her eyes swelled up. Whilst shooting *Desperate Housewives*, Nicollette Sheridan discovered that some of the flowers in Wisteria Lane triggered her hay fever. Other well-known sufferers include Kate Winslet, Cameron Diaz, Tiger Woods and Hugh Grant.

## Chapter 1

# About Hay Fever

This chapter gives you an overview of what hay fever is, as well as its symptoms and causes. It explains how the immune system is implicated in hay fever and discusses common allergens. It also considers other lifestyle, medical and environmental factors that may be involved and discusses how some of these have been blamed for the ever-increasing number of hay fever sufferers in the UK.

## 1. Learn about hay fever

### What is hay fever?

Hay fever, otherwise known as seasonal allergic rhinitis, is basically the immune system overreacting to the inhalation of pollen or fungal spores. Sufferers tend to be atopic, which means they are genetically predisposed to a number of allergic conditions – including eczema and asthma, as well as hay fever. Some people may suffer from hay fever symptoms practically all year round, depending on which pollen or spores they are allergic to. Some sufferers react to other allergens, such as house dust mites or pet dander (dead skin flakes).

Strictly speaking, this is not hay fever, but perennial allergic rhinitis, but I have included information about these allergens because the symptoms are the same and some people can suffer from both types. A recent study of nearly 1,000 people with hay fever showed that, on average, sufferers had severe symptoms for 15 working days each year. Some people find their symptoms are a minor, temporary nuisance, but for those whose symptoms are more persistent and severe, they can make life miserable, affecting school and work performance and enjoyment of leisure activities. Sufferers may also be reluctant to socialise, because they are embarrassed by the effects their hay fever symptoms have on their appearance.

## What are the symptoms?

Hay fever symptoms are similar to those associated with the common cold. The symptoms tend to come and go in cycles and can vary in severity. Studies show that people with multiple allergies tend to experience more extreme reactions. Research in Japan revealed that people with a house dust mite allergy who then go on to develop hay fever suffer more extreme symptoms than those who only have a single allergy. Hay fever can develop in childhood, or during the teenage years, and then disappear as the body becomes less sensitive to pollen. In some cases, it may return, or even develop for the first time, in middle age. However, its prevalence is highest among teenagers. When all age groups are taken into account, there is no gender bias for hay fever – although boys up to the age of ten are twice as likely to develop the condition as girls in that age group.

Common symptoms include:

**Sneezing** – a sign that the body is attempting to rid the nasal passages of the offending pollen.

**A runny or blocked nose** – an allergic response leads to increased mucus production and nasal congestion, as the blood vessels in the nose swell.

**Face pain and headache** – the sinus cavities can also become congested, causing pain just above the eyebrows, around the eyes and in the cheeks.

**A sore, itchy, nose and throat** – this is caused by the irritation and inflammation of the mucous membranes.

**Sore, itchy, gritty, watery eyes** – this is a result of irritation and inflammation, also known as 'allergic conjunctivitis', and the eyes attempting to flush out the pollen/spores.

**Itchy ears and palate** – this is a result of the body reacting to the allergen.

**An inability to concentrate** – having to deal with the symptoms can be distracting.

**Low mood** – coping with the uncomfortable symptoms and sleep deprivation can leave you feeling miserable.

**Disturbed sleep and tiredness** – symptoms like a blocked nose can disrupt sleep.

A small percentage of hay fever sufferers may develop additional symptoms such as:

**Pollen asthma** – some people develop this later on in the season, after a longer period of exposure to the allergen. Around one in five children with hay fever go on to develop asthma and four out of five asthma sufferers suffer from allergic rhinitis as well.

> **Important**
>
> If you develop a wheeze and a congested feeling that makes breathing difficult, you should visit your GP, as you may have pollen asthma.

**Sinusitis** – this is where the sinus cavities become inflamed or infected, causing pain. It can develop after repeated attacks of hay fever. Treatment with antibiotics may be necessary if there is an infection.

**Nasal polyps** – these are soft swellings in the nose that form as a result of an overgrowth of the lining. They can be caused by chronic inflammation through hay fever and other conditions.

**Nettle rash (urticaria)** – this may appear after coming into physical contact with the offending pollen.

**Atopic eczema** – this skin condition may be triggered by direct contact with allergens.

**Ear infection** – in children especially, hay fever often plays a part in middle ear infections.

## What else could it be?

If your streaming nose and eyes are accompanied by a temperature, it is likely that you are suffering from a cold or flu virus, rather than hay fever.

## What are the causes?

Atopy (allergy) is the root cause of hay fever. Other factors believed to be involved include chemical irritants, genetics, improved standards of hygiene, over-prescribing of antibiotics, paracetamol use in babies, the weather, global warming, pollution, diet and stress.

## Atopy (allergy)

A person who is atopic has an overly sensitive immune system that wrongly identifies substances like pollen as a threat to the body and then overreacts by producing too much of an antibody called Immunoglobulin E (IgE). Antibodies are proteins circulating in the bloodstream that are involved in the immune response. IgE binds to offending substances to enable other antibodies to remove them. This sets off a chain of chemical reactions in the body, known as inflammation.

## Sensitisation

An allergic reaction doesn't usually happen the first time you encounter an allergen. Your body has to 'learn' how to react, or become sensitised, to the allergen over a period of time. First of all, your body comes into contact with an allergen that the blood cells involved in your immune response perceive as a threat. Over the days or weeks that follow, your body produces allergic antibodies, which attach themselves to mast cells in your body's tissues. Mast cells produce a substance called histamine, which is designed to aid the removal of the offending agent and leads to inflammation and irritation. The next time your body encounters the allergen, your immune system immediately 'recognises' it as an 'enemy' and leaps into action, resulting in allergic symptoms, such as hay fever. In hay fever, histamine is released when pollen or fungal spores get into the eyes and are inhaled, resulting in swelling, itching and irritation in the mucous membranes in the eyes, nose, throat and sinuses, and increased mucus production.

## Common hay fever allergens

Common hay fever allergens include:

### Pollen

Pollen is a powder produced by flowering plants to fertilise other flowers. Pollen grains are so small they are invisible to the naked eye. They contain proteins that can trigger allergies. There are various pollens that can provoke symptoms. The most common culprit is grass pollen, with as many as 95 per cent of hay fever sufferers in the UK reacting to it. Around 25 per cent are allergic to birch pollen and another 20 per cent react to oak pollen. Pollen from weeds such as plantains, mugwort, nettles and docks also affects around 20 per cent of sufferers. Other culprits include the pollen from alder, hazel and horse chestnut trees. A person with hay fever can be allergic to just one, or several types of pollen. A recent survey of 928 hay fever sufferers revealed that 86 per cent were uncertain as to which type of pollen or spores they were allergic.

### Spores from fungi and moulds

Spores from fungi and moulds are a much less common cause of hay fever. In the UK, there are over 20 different moulds that can cause allergic reactions. Many can live indoors as well as outdoors, which means they can cause symptoms all year round, rather than just seasonal hay fever. Basidiospores (spores from mushrooms and toadstools, etc.) appear to provoke allergic reactions in around four per cent of sufferers.

## Other allergens

Other potential allergens include house dust mites, pet hair and dander, cut flowers, household cleaners, perfume and cosmetics, but these can cause symptoms all year round (perennial allergic rhinitis), rather than at particular times of the year as hay fever (seasonal allergic rhinitis) does.

### Chemical irritants

Exposure to chemical irritants such as cigarette smoke, air pollution, exhaust fumes, aerosol sprays, perfumes and paint fumes may cause irritant rhinitis. Whilst this form of rhinitis doesn't involve an allergic reaction, it can develop alongside allergic rhinitis (hay fever) and if it does, it is likely to be more severe.

### Genetics

Allergies tend to run in families. Children whose parents have allergies have an increased risk of developing them themselves, though they might appear in a different form. For example, a parent with asthma or eczema may have a child who has hay fever. Studies suggest that, despite some people inheriting a tendency towards developing allergies, they remain symptom-free, whilst other family members become allergic. A possible explanation for this is that exposure to allergens early on in life raises the likelihood of developing an allergy later on. Overall, 60 per cent of hay fever sufferers have a family history of atopy. The risk of developing hay fever is 30 per cent if one parent has a history of atopy, and 50 per cent if both parents are allergic.

## Improved hygiene

Some experts believe that improved hygiene standards in homes over the past few decades mean that many people have had less exposure to bacteria, which can help to develop a healthy immune system in childhood. As a result, their immune systems are underdeveloped, and overreact to non-harmful particles such as pollen or spores.

## Over-prescribing of antibiotics

Some experts cite the over-prescribing of antibiotics by GPs for the increasing incidence of hay fever. Antibiotics destroy 'good' bacteria, which disrupts the immune system and affects the immune response. This makes those who are genetically predisposed to allergies more likely to develop symptoms.

## Paracetamol in the first year of life

A study of 200,000 children concluded that giving paracetamol to babies just once a month during their first year increased their risk of developing hay fever by 48 per cent.

## The weather

The pollen count is usually higher on sunny days because more flowers open and release their pollen. As pollen levels rise, pollen is carried up into the air. On humid and windy days, pollen can spread further, which means that it can potentially cause more problems. Rain is actually good news for hay fever sufferers, because it washes pollen out of the atmosphere.

## Global warming

According to the Intergovernmental Panel on Climate Change, global warming is extending the hay fever season. The tree pollen seasons are starting earlier and grass and weed pollen seasons are lasting longer because of milder winters. Some experts predict that milder winters will enable ragweed – a major hay fever trigger in the US – to establish itself here in the UK. Also, trees are thought to produce more pollen in warmer temperatures.

## 'Litter-free' landscaping

A report in *New Scientist* magazine suggested that the current trend of planting male-only shrubs and trees in cities, to prevent the streets being littered with the pods, seeds and fruit that female plants produce, has contributed to the increase in hay fever, as it is male plants that produce pollen. With no female plants to trap the pollen and turn it into seed, pollen levels become unnaturally high.

## Pollution

Rising pollution levels over recent decades have also been blamed for the increasing number of hay fever sufferers – particularly in urban areas. An increase in the number of diesel-engine cars on the roads is thought to be a major factor. Pollen is thought to stick to heavy particles of diesel in the atmosphere, making it harder for it to disperse. As a result, pollen counts tend to be higher in urban areas. Pollutants from fossil fuels, such as nitrogen dioxide and sulphur dioxide, and other sources are also likely to be involved. The toxic particles are also believed to alter the chemical structure of pollens, making them even more likely to cause an allergic response. The nasal passages of hay fever sufferers are especially sensitive to the effects of pollutants, a condition known as 'nasal hyper-responsiveness'. Some researchers claim that increased $CO_2$ levels cause trees to mature earlier and produce more pollen. For more information about air pollution, as well as regional forecasts and bulletins, visit the UK National Air Quality Archive website (see the Directory).

## Diet

A poor diet that is lacking in essential vitamins and minerals may increase the risk of allergies. Some nutritional therapists believe that consuming too many dairy foods and sugary and refined foods leaves the body unable to deal with everyday substances like pollen and increases the production of mucus, which exacerbates symptoms.

## Stress

A stressful lifestyle seems to increase the risk of developing hay fever in the first place and may lead to more frequent and more severe attacks.

# Chapter 2

# Identify Your Allergens

One of the key things you can do to manage your hay fever symptoms is to identify the particular pollens and other allergens that trigger an attack. This chapter includes a questionnaire to help you to do this. Once you have identified your allergens, you can find ways to minimise your exposure to them. Conventional diagnostic tests and complementary or non-conventional tests that practitioners claim can identify allergies for hay fever are also discussed.

## 2. Complete the allergens questionnaire

1. Do you sneeze a lot and suffer from itchy and runny eyes and nose, but have a normal temperature (Around 37°C)? YES/NO
**YES** – you probably have hay fever. Go to question 2.
**NO** – you are likely to be suffering from a cold or flu virus – especially if your temperature is above 37°C.

2. Do you experience these symptoms from late May to mid-September, mainly early in the morning or late in the afternoon? YES/NO

**YES** – you are probably allergic to grass pollen.
**NO** – go to question 3.


3. Do your symptoms run from mid-March to mid-June? YES/NO
Do you suffer from an itchy mouth when you eat raw apples or stone fruits, such as peaches and plums? YES/NO
**YES** (to one or both questions) – you may be allergic to birch tree pollen. Apples and stone fruits have similar proteins to the birch tree and can therefore spark hay fever symptoms.
**NO** (to both questions) – go to question 4.


4. Do your symptoms appear in late summer? Are they fairly constant all day? YES/NO
**YES** (to first question or both) – it is likely you are allergic to weed pollen.
**NO** (to first question) – go to question 5.


5. Are your symptoms at their worst in the autumn and/or do you experience symptoms indoors? YES/NO
**YES** – (to one or both questions) you could be allergic to spores from outdoor or indoor moulds.
**NO** (to both questions) – go to question 6.


6. Do your symptoms occur all year round? YES/NO
**YES** – You may be allergic to numerous pollens and/or fungal spores, but it's also likely that other substances are to blame, such as spores from household moulds, house dust mites and pet dander.
**NO** – If you live in a big city go to question 7.


7. If you live in a big city – do your symptoms initially appear at the end of April/ beginning of May?

**YES** – You may be allergic to plane tree pollen – levels are particularly high in big cities, where there are a lot of plane trees. Your symptoms may also be exacerbated by pollution.

Once you have identified your allergens, see Chapter 3 for strategies to help you minimise their effects and Chapter 6 for details of medications that might prevent or treat your symptoms. The remaining chapters suggest dietary and lifestyle changes that may help you prevent or at least minimise your symptoms.

## Conventional allergy tests

Hay fever is usually easy to diagnose, but if you have symptoms all year round or particularly severe symptoms, or you are unsure about what you are allergic to, your GP may suggest a skin prick test or a RAST (Radio Allergo Sorbent Test) blood test.

A skin prick test is usually done first, because it is easy and quick to carry out. Suspected allergens, e.g. various pollens and fungal spores, are mixed with liquid to form a solution. A few drops of solution are applied to the skin, usually on the forearm, and then the area beneath is lightly pricked with a lancet to allow it to enter the skin. If the area reacts within about 10–15 minutes by becoming red, swollen and itchy, it confirms sensitivity to that substance. The person carrying out the test should then discuss the history of your symptoms, i.e. when and where they occur, as it is possible to be sensitised to a substance but not suffer an allergic reaction to it.

Your GP or allergy specialist may also do a RAST blood test to measure the levels of IgE antibodies in your blood. A blood sample is usually taken from a vein in the arm and sent off to a laboratory. The results are given as 'classes' ranging from zero (negative) to six (very high), or as the actual level. For example, a class three rating (high) indicates a level of IgE antibodies ranging from 3.50 KU/L (1,000 units per litre) to 17.49 KU/L. The interpretation of these results needs to be done carefully and your symptom history must also be taken into account before any conclusions can be drawn.

---

**Home tests**

You can buy home IgE tests, but Allergy UK does not recommend them because the results are not easy to read, so both false positive and false negative results are possible.

---

## Non-conventional allergy tests

These include Applied Kinesiology, which monitors changes in muscle strength, and Vega Testing, which detects disturbances in the body's electromagnetic fields. Hair analysis and pulse testing (Auricular Cardiac Reflex Method) are also used. However, none of these forms of allergy testing have been clinically proven, so they are generally deemed unreliable by conventional medical practitioners.

Chapter 3

# Practical Preventative Strategies

This chapter looks at practical preventative strategies to help you reduce the frequency and severity of your attacks. There is information about pollen and spores and details of when plants, trees, weeds, fungi and moulds release them, including their peak release periods. You will also find information about pollen counts and how to check them, as well as simple steps you can take to help reduce your exposure to other allergens and irritants that might exacerbate your symptoms.

## 3. Learn about pollen

Plants use pollen to reproduce – it carries male DNA to the female part of the flower. Many plants, including various trees and grasses, rely on the wind to carry their pollen. This means that the wind exerts a lot of influence on pollen levels. Plants release pollen twice each day – early in the morning and then late in the afternoon – but the wind can send pollen into the atmosphere at almost any time. Pollen counts tend to be at their highest early in the morning and in the evening on warm, dry, breezy days and at their lowest when the weather is wet and chilly. Pollens disappear after the first hard frost.

If there is little or no wind, pollen levels will be low. If the winds pick up, pollen levels will rise. A blustery wind will help to disperse the pollen, but it can also carry it further away. The count can depend on the direction of the wind. In the UK, the prevailing winds blow in a westerly direction: when the winds arrive from over the Atlantic they are practically pollen free, but as they travel over land, they pick up pollen. Hence, the west coast tends to have a much lower pollen count than the east coast. But if the winds come in from the east, the pollen count is higher on the west coast, as the wind travels across the land from the east, picking up pollen.

Pollen can be carried for long distances – pine pollen, probably from Norway, has been found on the UK's east coast. The pollen count in the Midlands has little to do with the direction the winds are coming from, because of its central position: winds bearing pollen travel in from all directions – so the counts in that region are often the highest in the UK. The pollen count in Derby one June reached 1,024 – a reading of 150 is considered very high. To make sure sufficient pollen reaches its intended destination, far more pollen grains are released than are needed and they have gradually evolved to enable them to stay in the air for longer – which is bad news for hay fever sufferers.

### Flower pollen

Flower pollen can also be a problem for hay fever sufferers. When my hay fever was at its worst, I would know there were cut flowers in a room before I'd even seen them, because my eyes and nose would react as soon as I walked in.

The majority of garden flowers bloom during the spring or summer. Roses are deemed to be low-allergen, because their pollen is so large it doesn't become airborne – those with the least fragrance are thought to produce the least pollen. Honeysuckle and orchids are also low-allergen flowers. Lilies are covered in powdery pollen – but as this is clearly visible, a non-allergic person can easily remove it, so they could be a good choice of cut flower for hay fever sufferers. Watch out for chrysanthemums and daisies, as these can be especially high in pollen.

## 4. Be aware of spores

Spores from fungi or moulds are a less common cause of hay fever. Spores are tiny grains from flowerless plants that are capable of forming new plants. The most likely culprits are spores from common species of fungi such as *Alternaria*, *Aspergillus* and *Cladosporium*. In the UK, there are over twenty types of moulds believed to cause allergic reactions. Many of these fungi can live indoors as well as outdoors – for example, types of *Aspergillus* are found in damp wallpaper and plaster, fireproofing, pipe lagging and air-conditioning systems and can be the cause of perennial rhinitis. Outside, *Aspergillus* can be found in damp rotting leaves, decaying vegetables and woodland.

### The pollen/spore seasons

This isn't an exact science – the timing and severity of both the pollen and spore seasons will vary from year to year, depending on the weather and also which part of the UK you are in. The start of the grass pollen season can vary by about a month, but tends to run from mid-May to mid-September. Weeds such as dock, nettle and plantain follow a similar pattern, while mugwort's pollen season starts about a month later. The pollen season for trees like alder, hazel and yew runs from January to April, whereas for birch, ash and plane trees, it is March to May. Birch pollen can also cause problems during the winter, as it cross-reacts with alder and hazel trees, which are part of the birch family. The season for oil seed rape and pine starts around March and ends about July. Common fungi such as *Cladosporium*, *Aspergillus* and *Alternaria* release spores from September to March, whereas spores from mushrooms and toadstools (basidiospores) are released from September to December. The concentrations of *Aspergillus* spores are thought to be fairly low compared to other moulds. Each of these plants/moulds has a peak period of pollen/spore release (except for *Aspergillus*, whose spore levels remain fairly constant), which tends to correspond with the highest numbers of people reporting symptoms. Peak levels are usually reached later in the north of the UK than in the south because of the slightly cooler climate there.

## The pollen/spore calendar

Having an awareness of the peak pollen/spore release periods will enable you to implement your prevention and treatment strategies at the right time.

The table below gives a guide to the peak periods of pollen/spore release in the UK.

| Month | Tree/Grass/Weed/Fungus/Mould |
|-------|------------------------------|
| January | alder, hazel, willow |
| February | alder, hazel, yew |
| March | alder, elm, hazel, poplar, willow, yew |
| April | alder, ash, birch, oak, yew, elm, willow, plane |
| May | grass (inc. cocksfoot, rye & timothy), pine, oil seed rape and plane |
| June | dock, grass (inc. cocksfoot, rye & timothy), lime, nettle, pine, plantain |
| July | grass (inc. cocksfoot, rye & timothy), mugwort, nettle |
| August | mugwort |
| September | basidiospores, Alternaria, Cladosporium |
| October | basidiospores |
| November | basidiospores |

For a more detailed pollen and fungal spore calendar visit www.pollenforecast.org (see Directory), or for a Generalised UK Pollen and Fungal Spores Calendar visit www.devoninformation.com.

## 5. Check the pollen/spore counts

The pollen count is the average number of pollen grains per cubic metre of air over a period of 24 hours. The counts given are usually for grass, birch and nettles. A low count is less than 30 pollen grains per cubic metre of air, which won't cause symptoms in the majority of sufferers – except in people who are unusually sensitive. A count of

30 to 49 is moderate, but could cause symptoms in some people; 50 to 149 is high; 150 to 499 is very high; and over 500 is exceedingly high. A high to very high pollen count will cause problems for most hay fever sufferers.

Spores are much smaller than pollen grains and far more are released into the atmosphere. Less than 1,000 fungal spores is classed as a very low count; 1,000 to 4,999 is low; 5,000 to 19,999 is moderate; and 20,000 to 50,000 is high. A count of 50,000 and above is deemed very high.

These counts are useful because they show when the different pollen/spore seasons start, which can help you assess whether your symptoms are due to hay fever or not and to determine the best time to start taking preventative medications and when to stop. For further information about pollen and spores, visit NPARU's website (see Directory). If you check the pollen and spore forecast on a daily basis, you will be able to plan activities accordingly – visit www.pollenforecast.org. The BBC also gives information on pollen and spore counts during weather bulletins and in their online local weather forecasts – go to www.bbc.co.uk/weather. If you have a mobile on which you can access the Internet, you can find out about pollen levels where you are by texting 'WEATHER' to 81010. This will give you a link to the BBC's online weather forecasts.

## 6. Reduce your exposure to pollen/spores

Below are some simple steps you can take to reduce your exposure to pollen/spores – particularly when you know a high count is forecast and during peak pollen release times (7 a.m. to 10 a.m. and 4 p.m. to 7 p.m.) and peak spore release times (1 p.m. to 5 p.m.).

- Smear vaseline around and just inside your nostrils to form a barrier that traps pollen/spores.

- Try wearing nasal filters (see Useful Products). These are discreet plastic devices worn inside the nostrils. There is evidence that they can help to reduce hay fever symptoms.

- Wear wraparound sunglasses to protect your eyes from pollen/spores and sunlight, which can trigger sneezing.

- Sniff cool water up your nose then spit it out, to flush pollen/spores from your nasal passages.

- Swap contact lenses for glasses, or choose daily or disposable types, as pollen/spores can collect on them.

- Avoid wearing mascara as pollen/spores stick to it – have your eyelashes dyed instead.

- Rinse pollen/spores from sore, irritated eyes using chilled, distilled water.

- Place a cold, used tea bag on each eye to soothe them and relieve itching.

- Keep your windows closed, or consider buying an air-purifying unit (see Directory and Useful Products).

- Dry washing indoors rather than outside, where pollen/spores will stick to it.

- Pets can carry pollen/spores in their fur – ask a family member to groom or wash them when they have been outdoors.

- Wipe down surfaces and vacuum regularly, preferably using a cleaner with a HEPA (High Efficiency Particulate Arresting) filter, to keep your home pollen/spore free.

- Avoid mowing the lawn or gardening, or wear a pollen mask to prevent pollen/spore inhalation through your nose and mouth (see Useful Products).

- Drive with your car windows closed. Use the air conditioning system on 're-circulate' mode instead and consider installing an in-car air filter, air purifier, or pollen filter.

- After being outdoors, change your clothes and launder them. Take a bath or shower to rinse away pollen/spores from your hair and body.

- In the autumn, keep your garden clear of leaves and other debris that can harbour spores.

- Avoid woodland walks in damp conditions, or among rotting leaves where moulds grow.

- Consider using an air purifier, air filter, or air conditioner to reduce pollen and spore levels in your home (See Useful Products, and Allergy UK in the Directory).

## Avoiding allergens in the home

Moulds can also exist indoors. And, as a hay fever sufferer, it's possible that you are allergic to other substances as well as, or rather than, pollen and mould spores. Dust mites and pet dander are common indoor allergens that can also cause problems.

## 7. Manage mould

Mould can release thousands of microscopic spores into the atmosphere, which can cause allergic rhinitis, so it's important to prevent it from developing around your home. Moulds, such as those from the *Cladosporium* and *Aspergillus* families, favour the damp, musty conditions often found in kitchens and bathrooms and on window frames. Indoor levels of *Cladosporium* spores tend to correspond with the levels outdoors, as they are easily carried in the air. To prevent mould, follow the advice given below regarding house dust mites. A solution containing equal amounts of white vinegar and water is excellent for the safe removal of mould around the home. To prevent mould growing on the soil in house plant pots, cover with a layer of pea shingle (fine gravel). Real Christmas trees can harbour mould and cause symptoms over the festive period – especially if you spray them with water to prevent needle drop. If you're affected, consider having an artificial tree.

## 8. Control dust mites

House dust mites live on the human dead skin cells found in household dust. The waste matter from house dust mites can be a hay fever trigger for some people.

### Clean up
Clean rooms thoroughly each week: wipe floors, furniture, window sills and frames and even door tops with a damp cloth to remove dust. Use a vacuum cleaner with a HEPA filter.

### Go carpet-free
Carpet fibres can harbour dust and therefore make an ideal home for dust mites, making hard floors a better alternative; the current trend for wooden and tiled floors is beneficial for perennial allergic rhinitis sufferers, because dust and dirt are more visible and they're easier to keep clean.

### Curtain call
Use blinds rather than curtains, as they're easier to keep dust-free. However, avoid venetian blinds, as they tend to gather dust and are harder to clean. Roman, roller, pleated and vertical blinds are relatively easy to keep dust-free – try using the brush attachment on your vacuum cleaner.

### Cuddly toy cooler
Children's cuddly toys are an ideal home for dust mites. Dust mites die at temperatures above 60°C and below 0°C (freezing), so one way of killing them is to place soft toys in a plastic bag and then

put them in the freezer. Leave them there for at least six hours, or overnight, then wash afterwards to remove any dead mites and their droppings.

## Blitz your bedding

The dust mite's favourite haunt is in your bedding. Your mattress alone can harbour up to three million dust mites. Your pillow can double its weight in six months as dust mites accumulate inside it. To reduce numbers, pull back the bedclothes every morning and allow the mattress to air for at least an hour – preferably with the windows open. Wash sheets, duvet covers and pillowcases once a week at 60°C. Vacuum the mattress before replacing the bedding. Wash duvets and pillows as often as possible. Those made from synthetic fibres are easier to wash than those with feathers. Where possible, hang bedding outside to dry. You can also buy mite-resistant pillows and duvets and mite-resistant covers for your mattress and duvet. Allergy UK provides a list of approved stockists (see Directory).

## Check your home's humidity

Mites like warm, damp conditions. To keep them at bay, ensure your home's humidity level stays between 45 and 55 per cent. If you suspect the atmosphere in your home is too damp, use a hygrometer, a device that measures humidity, to check the amount of moisture in the air. Opening your windows every day will help to reduce humidity. Keeping doors shut when cooking and showering or taking a bath and using extractor fans can help. If you dry laundry in a tumble dryer, make sure it is vented to the outside, or use a condenser drier. Or you can use a dehumidifier to achieve the ideal humidity level. For details of where you can buy a compact thermo-hygrometer suitable for domestic use, see the Useful Products section. For further information about house dust mites and how to control them, visit www.housedustmite.org.

## 9. Clear up pet hair/dander

Around ten million people in the UK find that pet hair or dander (skin flakes) trigger allergies, including hay fever-type symptoms. If you're a pet owner, this can make life very difficult. There are products available that are aimed at removing allergens from pets' coats, which usually take the form of lotions or shampoos that are rubbed into the fur and then wiped, or rinsed off, taking the allergens with them. A HEPA air purifier may also help (see Useful Products).

## 10. Clean your home naturally

Instead of using products that are laden with chemicals, choose eco-friendly cleaners based on natural ingredients, such as those in the Ecover range – for further details go to the Useful Products section. Supermarkets also often produce their own plant-based ranges. Alternatively, you can make your own, using items from your kitchen cupboard such as vinegar, lemons, salt and bicarbonate of soda.

**Natural whitener**
Borax (a natural mineral salt containing boron) can be used as a gentle alternative to bleach. To remove stains on white cotton or linen, apply directly then rinse. Soak coloured fabrics in a weak solution of borax – made by adding 20 g (one tablespoon) to 500 ml of water – for no longer than 15 minutes. For an all-purpose household cleaner

and disinfectant, mix one teaspoon of borax with two tablespoons of white vinegar and one litre of hot water.

---

### Household cleaners

Many chemical-based household cleaners contain irritants and allergens that may exacerbate hay fever symptoms. In a recent study by the World Wildlife Fund involving 47 volunteers, between 13 and 54 out of 101 man-made chemicals were detected in individual volunteers' bodies. Many of these were found to have come from household cleaning products and were identified as harmful.

---

## Soda solution

Bicarbonate of soda is cheap and very versatile. Mixed with water, it forms an alkaline solution that helps dissolve dirt and grease and neutralise smells. It can be used on carpets to remove stains. To clean a smelly drain, sprinkle one cupful of bicarbonate of soda into it, then slowly pour one cup of white vinegar down. The resulting foam removes grease and deodorises. Sprinkled on a damp cloth, bicarbonate of soda acts as a mild abrasive that removes marks from surfaces without scratching them. Use it in this way on plastic, porcelain, glass, tiles and stainless steel. Use it in the bathroom to clean the bath and washbasin and in the kitchen to clean appliances. Fill a small container with bicarbonate and leave in the fridge to absorb odours. Stir it occasionally and replace every three months or so. To clean and freshen your dishwasher, add one cup of bicarbonate and run it on the rinse cycle whilst empty. For difficult stains, mix with a little water to make a paste, apply and leave for a few minutes before rinsing off. Silver emerges clean and shiny when cleaned in this way.

## Lemon freshener

Lemons contain citric acid, which makes them great natural cleaners, with bleaching, antiseptic, antibacterial and degreasing qualities. Half a lemon makes a great bath and washbasin cleaner. Use it on the taps to remove limescale and leave them gleaming. Buff them afterwards with a dry cloth. To clean copper and brass, dip half a lemon into salt and rub. Rinse well immediately to prevent discolouration. Lemon is also a natural bleach. To brighten clothing and bed linen, soak them in a bucket of water to which you've added the juice of a lemon. Leave overnight before washing as normal. Lemon also deodorises. To clean the microwave and remove food smells, place a couple of slices of lemon into a microwaveable bowl containing water. Microwave for a couple of minutes, then wipe using kitchen roll or a clean cloth. To keep your fridge fresh, place a couple of slices of lemon inside.

## Natural polish

Olive oil is an excellent natural substitute for commercial furniture polish. Mix a cup of ordinary olive oil with the juice of one lemon and pour it into a spray bottle. To polish wooden surfaces, spray a little on to the surface and rub. The lemon juice cuts through the dirt, whilst the olive oil shines and protects the wood. Use a dry cloth to remove the excess oil and buff to a shine. Use sparingly, as excessive amounts of oil could leave the surface feeling sticky. Olive oil is also good for removing fingerprints from stainless steel surfaces and cooking utensils. Simply sprinkle a little on some kitchen roll and buff.

## Versatile vinegar

Vinegar is a dilute solution of acetic acid that cuts through grease, deodorises and is mildly disinfectant. White vinegar is the best type to use around your home, as it doesn't have a strong smell. Mix equal amounts of white vinegar and water in a spray bottle and use as a general cleaner. It's especially good on tiles and kitchen worktops. For a fresh fragrance, add a few drops of lemongrass, bergamot or geranium essential oils. For difficult stains, use warm water. Cover the stain with the vinegar solution and leave for ten minutes before wiping off. White vinegar also makes a great window cleaner – use half a cup in a litre of warm water. Spray onto your window and then remove and buff with crumpled newspapers to avoid streaking.

Vinegar is a good descaler. To clean a showerhead, simply remove it and soak in undiluted vinegar. To remove limescale from your kettle, fill with vinegar and leave overnight. Pour the liquid out the next day and rinse well before using. To descale taps, soak a few paper towels in white vinegar. Wrap them around the taps, and cover with plastic bags held in place with elastic bands. Leave for a few hours before rinsing and buffing with a dry cloth.

## Ketchup cleaner

If you've run out of vinegar, tomato ketchup makes a good, if slightly messy, substitute, as it contains acetic acid. It's especially recommended for cleaning copper and brass.

## Natural disinfectant and fungicide

Australian tea tree oil – *Melaleuca alternifolia* – is an excellent natural disinfectant and fungicide. For a general-purpose disinfectant solution, mix 10 ml (two teaspoons) of tea tree oil with two cups of water. To remove and reduce mould and mildew growth, use the solution in a spray bottle and squirt on the affected areas. Leave for a few minutes and then rinse with warm, soapy water. To keep shower curtains mildew-free and to remove strong mildew smells from fabrics, add a few drops of tea tree oil to your usual washing powder.

## 11. Make your home a smoke-free zone

Cigarettes contain many chemicals that could exacerbate hay fever symptoms, especially those affecting the eyes. Smoking also uses up vitamin C – low levels are thought to increase the risk of allergies. Avoid smoky areas and, if you smoke, consider giving up.

### Perfume problems

Perfumes may also irritate the nasal passages and exacerbate symptoms, and some may provoke allergic responses in sensitive individuals. Avoid strong perfumes in general and, once you've identified your own particular culprits, try to avoid them. Perfume oils, which are free of alcohol and usually contain fewer chemicals, may be less irritating than conventional alcohol-based fragrances. The Body Shop sells a range of perfume oils.

**Chapter 4**

# The Food Factor

A healthy, balanced diet with few refined foods and plenty of fruit, vegetables, oily fish, nuts and seeds, may help to keep your immune system functioning normally and prevent hay fever symptoms developing. Naturopath Roger Newman Turner, a trustee of the Research Council for Complementary Medicine, said recently that, during nearly 40 years of practice, he had discovered that diet plays a very important role in the management of hay fever. He added: 'Most of my hay fever patients have been able to reduce the severity of their symptoms and, in some cases, eradicate the condition.' This chapter looks at how your diet may be implicated in your hay fever symptoms and discusses the foods and supplements that could help.

Warning: an exclusion diet should only be undertaken under the supervision of a dietician, or other suitably qualified medical professional, as cutting out whole food groups can result in nutritional deficiencies.

## 12. Cut back on dairy products

Some experts, including Roger Newman Turner, believe that cutting back on dairy products can help to relieve hay fever symptoms by reducing the amount of mucus produced. You could try removing these foods for a couple of weeks and see if there is any improvement in your symptoms. However, calcium is essential for a healthy nervous system, as well as strong bones and teeth, so if you decide to stop eating dairy products in the long term, you need to ensure your diet contains alternative sources of this important mineral. Non-dairy sources of calcium include tinned sardines eaten with the bones, apricots, dates, figs, almonds, brazil nuts, seeds, green leafy vegetables, watercress, leeks, tofu and soya – soya milk usually has added calcium. Alternatively, or as an added insurance, you could consider taking a calcium supplement. Supplements containing calcium carbonate may increase your risk of developing kidney stones. Instead, choose one containing calcium citrate, which is more easily absorbed – such as Solgar Calcium Citrate with vitamin D.

## 13. Consider eating less wheat

Wheat is another food that some nutritionists claim can make hay fever symptoms worse. One theory is that because this originates from a grass product, some hay fever sufferers become hypersensitive to the proteins in it. However, there is no clinical evidence that this is the case. Intensive farming practices mean that wheat is now higher in gluten than in the past, and gluten is thought to irritate the gut and increase the production of mucus in some people. You could try excluding wheat products for a month to see if your hay fever symptoms improve. Eat rye breads, crackers and crisp breads, oats and oat cakes, gluten-free flours, brown rice, millet, quinoa and buckwheat instead.

## 14. Eat foods high in essential fatty acids

Eat oily fish, such as salmon, mackerel and sardines, and nuts and seeds and their oils, e.g. sunflower and flaxseed oils. These are rich in omega-3 and omega-6 essential fatty acids, which contain hormone-like substances called prostaglandins that have anti-inflammatory properties and may help to reduce hay fever symptoms. Some nutritionists advise at least three servings of oily fish each week. If you dislike it, consider taking a fish oil supplement. Nuts and seeds also contain zinc, which is thought to strengthen the immune system.

### Vitamin A and D intake

Don't take fish oil supplements alongside a multivitamin, as they both contain vitamins A and D, which are fat soluble. This means that any excess is stored in the liver. Too much of these vitamins can be harmful.

## 15. Eat antioxidant-rich fruit and vegetables

Eating plenty of fruit and vegetables will ensure that your diet is high in antioxidants such as beta-carotene and vitamins C and E. Antioxidants are thought to neutralise the effects of pollution and to help maintain a healthy immune system. According to Roger

Newman Turner, a diet based on raw fruit and vegetables reduces inflammation in the body. Vitamin C, which is found mainly in citrus fruits, berries and green vegetables such as broccoli and cabbage, is thought to have antihistamine effects. The body turns beta-carotene into vitamin A, which keeps the mucous membranes healthy. Yellow and orange fruits and vegetables such as apricots, cantaloupe melons, butternut squash, carrots, orange and yellow peppers, and sweet potatoes, are rich in beta-carotene. Vitamin E is found in avocados, eggs, oily fish, sweet potatoes, nuts and seeds, olive oil and wheatgerm. A recent study at the Harvard Medical School suggested that a diet rich in these foods helps to prevent the development of hay fever symptoms.

## Hay fever and oral allergy syndrome

A recent report from Allergy UK highlighted how certain fruits, vegetables, nuts and spices can occasionally provoke an allergic reaction when eaten by some hay fever sufferers – especially those with an allergy to birch pollen. The report suggested that this is because they contain similar proteins to those found in pollens from trees (especially birch), grasses and weeds. The main fruits that can cause such problems are raw apples, peaches, pears and cherries and, to a lesser degree, apricots, mangoes, kiwis, oranges, plums, nectarines and lychees. Carrots and celery are the vegetables most likely to cause a reaction. Peppers, raw potatoes, raw tomatoes and raw onions may also affect some sufferers. Hazlenuts are another common culprit and other nuts such as Brazil nuts, peanuts, walnuts and almonds can affect some people. Spices such as coriander, aniseed and caraway seed may also provoke a reaction. The symptoms are usually mild and may include itching, tingling and swelling inside and around the mouth, although the throat can sometimes also be affected. Allergy UK recommends rinsing the mouth with plain water and taking an antihistamine.

If you believe you are affected, ask your GP to arrange an allergy test. If your suspicions are confirmed, you can then avoid the culprit/s. In severe cases, an EpiPen (adrenaline injector) may be prescribed.

Caution: If you experience breathing difficulties, or your throat feels like it's closing up, ring an ambulance immediately and use your EpiPen if you have one. For more information, visit Allergy UK's website (see the Directory).

## 16. Choose low-GI foods

Some nutritionists believe that low blood sugar is implicated in allergies. Missing meals and eating the wrong types of foods can lead to low blood sugar, which they claim leaves the body unable to cope with everyday substances like pollen and house dust mites. Eating regularly, which means never going for longer than four hours without food and choosing foods with a low Glycaemic Index (GI), can help to keep the blood sugar steady.

The GI is a measure of the rate at which a food raises the level of sugar in the blood. Refined carbohydrates such as white bread, pastries, sugary drinks and sweets convert easily into glucose, causing your blood sugar to rise rapidly, which means they have a high GI. Some nutritional therapists claim that these foods also increase mucus production. Carbohydrates such as multigrain bread, porridge, sweet potatoes, pasta and basmati or brown rice take longer to digest and cause your blood glucose to rise slowly and remain steady for a longer period of time, so they have a low GI.

For a low-GI diet:

◯ Replace all refined carbohydrates such as white bread, biscuits, pastries and sweets with wholegrains.

◯ Eat lots of fruit and vegetables, low-fat yogurts and cheeses, and skimmed/semi-skimmed milk.

◯ Include small amounts of nuts, fish and lean meat.

◯ Leave the skins on potatoes so that they take longer to digest. New potatoes, boiled in their skins, have the lowest GI.

◯ As well as eating regular meals, have healthy snacks such as fresh fruit, oat cakes, natural yogurt, or a small handful of nuts or seeds.

This type of diet will also help you manage your weight healthily without resorting to strict dieting, which could contribute to the development of hay fever symptoms, especially if you miss meals in an effort to lose weight. It may also help to reduce the amount of mucus your body produces, which may in turn help to reduce hay fever symptoms.

## 17. Drink green tea

Green tea is rich in powerful antioxidants, known as catechins, which are thought to have a natural antihistamine effect and help maintain a healthy immune system. Drinking two to three cups of green tea every day, especially during the hay fever season, may help to keep symptoms at bay.

### Try an old folk remedy

Sipping cider vinegar is an old folk remedy for hay fever. According to an American doctor called Deforest Clinton Jarvis, author of *Folk Medicine: A famous doctor's guide to folk medicine practices of Vermont – the nature secrets of honey, apple cider vinegar and foods for good health*, apple cider vinegar contains vitamins, minerals and enzymes that are beneficial to health. There is only anecdotal evidence that it works, but I believe it is still worth trying. Add one to two tablespoons to a glass of water and drink two to three times a day. If you dislike the taste, try adding one teaspoon of honey, or stir it into a glass of apple or other fruit juice.

## 18. Have a spoonful of honey

Taking one tablespoon of local honey daily from around one month before the start of the hay fever season is reported to help reduce attacks. It's claimed that the tiny amounts of grass and tree pollen picked up by bees as they visit flowers for nectar find their way into the honey they produce and have a desensitising effect. The honey needs to have been produced within a ten-mile radius of where you live and work to ensure that you develop immunity to the pollen to which you are usually exposed. Although these claims aren't backed up by clinical evidence, there is anecdotal evidence that this works.

## 19. Boost your beneficial bacteria

Probiotics are beneficial bacteria strains such as *Lactobacillus*, *Bifidobacteria* and *Acidophilus*, which are believed to help boost the immune system. Popular brands include the probiotic drinks Yakult and Actimel, and Activia yogurts.

Research published in the journal *Clinical & Experimental Allergy* suggested that probiotics may change the way hay fever sufferers' immune systems react to grass pollen.

Scientists from the Institute of Food Research (IFR) in the UK randomly gave ten hay fever sufferers either a probiotic yoghurt drink containing *Lactobacillus casei shirota* or a placebo (a yoghurt drink without probiotic bacteria) every day for five months. After five months, the hay fever sufferers who had drunk the probiotic yoghurt drink every day had significantly lower levels of IgE and other chemicals linked to allergies than the sufferers who were given the placebo. The researchers also reported that those in the probiotic group had higher levels of another type of antibody called immunoglobulin G (IgG), which provides protection against allergic reactions.

Although this study was only small, the researchers stated they were 'fascinated to discover a response' and that they expected to confirm these results in the future with a larger study. They also hoped to discover whether the lower levels of IgE were directly linked to the reduction in hay fever symptoms amongst participants.

If you want to add probiotics to your diet to determine whether they can help your symptoms, you could either try one of the many probiotic drinks on the market or eat natural or fruit-flavoured bio yogurt. Many of these drinks are high in sugar, so look out for 'light' versions. Fruit-flavoured yogurts also tend to have added sugar, whereas natural yogurt doesn't. You could also try probiotic supplements, which usually contain higher doses of probiotics and are enteric-coated so that more 'good' bacteria are likely to survive the acids in your stomach and reach your intestines, where they can grow and multiply. You will probably need to take probiotics every day for at least a month before you notice any benefits.

### Prebiotics

Some probiotic supplements have prebiotics added – these are natural sugars that feed 'good' bacteria and encourage them to multiply. They are usually listed as either *inulin* (found in vegetables) or *fructo-oligosaccharrides* (found in fruit). You can boost your intake of prebiotics by eating foods like artichokes, leeks, celery, cucumber and tomatoes.

## 20. Eat foods containing quercetin

Eating foods like red onions, berries, red grapes and red apples may help because they contain quercetin, an antioxidant that has been found to help prevent hay fever. Quercetin is thought to work by preventing the release of histamine. It's also believed to stabilise cell membranes, so that they are less likely to react to allergens like pollen.

## 21. Go for garlic

Garlic also contains quercetin and sulphur compounds called diallyl sulphides and allicin, which are thought to boost the immune system, reduce mucus and have anti-inflammatory properties.

## 22. Soothe symptoms with supplements

Supplements are often controversial, with some recent research claiming that isolated substances don't provide the same benefits that nutrients found in foods do. However, if you find it difficult to eat a balanced diet every day, supplements represent a convenient means of ensuring an adequate intake of vitamins and minerals, or including beneficial herbs in a palatable form. Often there is anecdotal evidence but no, or insufficient, conclusive evidence that a supplement works. This doesn't necessarily mean that it's ineffective – often it's just that the research hasn't been done. Sometimes, the type of research undertaken gives results that are deemed inconclusive. For example, if an uncontrolled study is carried out with only one group of participants and no comparison group taking a different treatment, or having no treatment at all, the results may be unreliable, because any improvement may happen purely because a participant expects it to, rather than because of the treatment itself. This is known as the 'placebo effect'.

A Traditional Herbal Medicines Registration Scheme currently exists, but unregistered herbal products can still be sold – providing they are marketed as food supplements and comply with certain legal requirements. This means that there is no absolute guarantee of their content and quality. With EU legislation that will come into force in April 2011, all herbal medicines will be required to have either a traditional herbal medicine registration or a product licence.

Registered herbal medicines must meet specific standards of safety and quality and carry agreed indications for their use. They are identified by the prefix THR, followed by a nine-digit number.

Licensed herbal medicines, like any other medicine, are required to demonstrate safety, quality and effectiveness and provide guidelines on safe usage. These are identified by a nine-digit number, prefixed with the letters PL. In the meantime, always buy products from a reputable company and, if in doubt, check with your GP or pharmacist. The government agency the Medicines and Healthcare products Regulatory Agency (MHRA) lists herbal products currently registered under the Traditional Herbal Medicines Registration Scheme, along with information sheets on their safe use. Its contact details can be found in the Directory at the end of this book.

It is best to start taking herbal and other supplements at least one month before you expect your symptoms to start, in order to allow their anti-allergic properties to build up in your system. Details of products containing the herbs listed below can be found in the Useful Products section.

> ### Inform your GP
>
> Always inform your GP if you are taking a herbal supplement, as some can make conventional drugs less effective.

## Beta glucans

Beta glucans are plant nutrients found in naturally occurring yeasts on fruits and grains that are thought to normalise the immune system, thereby reducing the risk of it overreacting to harmless substances like pollen. Dr Paul Clayton, a medical pharmacologist, blames the widespread use of fungicides, ultra-filtration of wines and beers and modern bread-making methods for a lack of beta glucans in our diets. He claims this shortage of beta glucans is one of the factors involved in the increase in allergies like hay fever and recommends eating organic vegetables and home-made bread. Alternatively, you can buy a beta glucans supplement.

## Butterbur

Butterbur is a plant from the daisy family with anti-inflammatory properties. Studies suggest it is as effective in relieving hay fever symptoms as antihistamines like cetirizine and fexofenadine, but has the added benefit of not causing drowsiness. A Swiss study found that when hay fever sufferers took 50 mg of butterbur daily, they had improved nasal air flow and their sneezing, itching and conjunctivitis were relieved. It is believed to work by releasing petasins, which are thought to relax the muscles and blood vessels. Make sure that the product you choose is free from alkaloid compounds, as these can cause liver damage.

## Calming chamomile

Chamomile contains anti-inflammatory agents and there is anecdotal evidence that drinking chamomile tea regularly helps to soothe the symptoms of hay fever. Chamomile tea bags are widely available – after use and once cooled they can be placed on your closed eyes to reduce puffiness and soreness. You can also make your own tea. Chamomile can be grown in a sunny spot, in pots or in the garden. Pick the flowers whilst in full bloom and hang them upside down in small bunches in a well-ventilated warm room until they are crisp and completely dry. Store the dried flowers in an airtight jar. To make a cup of chamomile tea, pour boiling water over one tablespoon of the dried flowers, cover and leave to stand for five to ten minutes. Strain, add honey to taste and drink whilst hot. Chamomile tea has a distinctive, apple-like flavour. If you dislike the taste, try adding two or three tea bags to a hot bath to enjoy the benefits without having to drink the tea.

### Easy infusion

Use a coffee cafetière to make a herbal infusion quickly and easily. Place the herbs/flowers in the cafetière and add boiling water. Replace the lid. Leave to brew, then press down the plunger and pour.

## Elder

Elder (sambucus) is a sub-tropical shrub that has traditionally been used by herbalists to treat respiratory conditions. Both the flowers and berries are thought to have anti-inflammatory and immune-boosting properties. According to a study published in the *Journal of International Medical Research*, the berries may ease nasal congestion and a runny nose. The flowers are thought to strengthen the respiratory tract. Herbalists recommend that you start taking elderberries or elderflowers as an infusion or tincture before the hay fever season starts, in order to reduce the frequency and severity of attacks. When the flowers appear in June/July, you can make your own infusion by adding two fresh elderflower heads or 10 g (two teaspoons) of dried elderflowers to a cup of boiling water.

Pick newly opened flowers on a warm, dry day from a traffic-free area. Shake well to remove any insects and remove stalks before using. Use fresh, or dry them by spreading them out on a tray in a warm spot. Store them in airtight glass jars in a cool dark place for up to one year.

### Eyebright (*Euphrasia officinalis*)

Eyebright is an alpine herb that is believed to have anti-inflammatory properties and to help soothe both the eyes and mucous membranes. David Hoffman, author of *The Herbal Handbook: A User's Guide to Medical Herbalism*, says that, when taken internally, eyebright is an effective anti-catarrhal and may also act as a decongestant. It's available both in eye drops and as a homeopathic remedy (see Help yourself with homeopathy on page 107).

### Guduchi (*Tinospora cordifolia*)

A herb used in Ayurvedic medicine for various conditions and to boost immune function. In one double-blind study, the majority of hay fever sufferers who were given 300 mg of a standardised extract three times daily for eight weeks reported a significant improvement in symptoms like sneezing, runny nose, nasal congestion and nasal itching.

## Nettle

This common weed has traditionally been used to treat hay fever. Nettles contain histamine and formic acid, as well as vitamins and minerals. Supplements containing dried nettle extract have been shown to curb the release of chemicals that trigger hay fever symptoms. Some studies report an improvement in symptoms. You could also try drinking nettle tea. Nettle tea bags are quite widely available, or you can make your own infusion: pick young leaves (wearing gloves) and add about 15 g (3 teaspoons) to one cup of boiling water.

## Pycnogenol

Taking a pycnogenol supplement may cut hay fever symptoms and help breathing by reducing the amount of histamines released and relaxing constricted blood vessels. Pycnogenol is extracted from the bark of French maritime pine. According to a study published in *Phytotherapy Research*, a supplement containing pycnogonel reduced the production of histamines caused by airborne allergens by 70 per cent.

## Sponge cucumber (*Luffa operculata*)

Sponge cucumber is a tropical plant that appears to act as a natural antihistamine. It can reduce symptoms like sneezing, itchy, runny eyes and nose, and a blocked or stuffy nose, without causing the drowsiness and fatigue that many medications do. A recent Dutch study found that 75 per cent of participants with hay fever reported a big reduction in symptoms when taking a sponge cucumber supplement. Products containing extracts from this plant include nasal sprays and tablets.

## Vitamin C

Vitamin C is essential for a healthy immune system and may help to reduce hay fever symptoms. One study, published in *Ear, Nose And Throat Journal*, reported that vitamin C reduced hay fever symptoms in 74 per cent of patients. Other studies suggest that taking 500 mg of vitamin C a day and gradually increasing the dose to 2 g can reduce histamine levels in the blood by as much as 40 per cent. As a result, sensitivity to allergens, wheezing and mucus production are reduced. According to the 'Food Doctor' Ian Marber, a low intake of this vitamin may lead to a build-up of histamine in the bloodstream and cause attacks of hay fever. Some nutritionists recommend taking one 500-mg tablet four times daily, as one large dose can cause diarrhoea in some people.

## Vitamin E

Some research suggests that vitamin E can help to ease a blocked or runny nose when it is taken alongside other hay fever treatments.

## 23. Consider nutritional therapists' advice

Ian Marber the 'Food Doctor' recommends eating ginger, saying that it slows down the production of histamine. Ginger is anti-inflammatory and helps to relieve nasal congestion. Try taking it as a tea, made by pouring boiling water over three or four thin slices of peeled ginger root. Sweeten to taste with honey. He also suggests taking a bromelain supplement, claiming it is useful for boosting anti-inflammatory prostaglandins.

Patrick Holford, another leading nutritional therapist, advises taking vitamin B6 and zinc supplements to balance histamine levels and keep the immune system healthy. For severe symptoms, he recommends taking 500 mg of the amino acid methionine, 400 mg of calcium (for their antihistamine effects) and 500 mg of vitamin B5, twice daily. If your symptoms are particularly troublesome, he advocates taking a 500 mg quercetin supplement three times daily, dropping down to once a day once they are under control.

## Chapter 5

# Hay Fever and Emotions

This chapter looks at how stress may affect the immune response and increase the frequency and severity of attacks. Suffering from hay fever can be stressful – it can have a huge impact on your work, family and social life. Stress management and relaxation techniques that may not only help to prevent attacks, but also help you to cope during one, are included.

## What is stress?

Stress is basically the way the mind and body respond to situations and pressures that leave us feeling inadequate or unable to cope. One person may cope well in a situation that another might find stressful: it's all down to the individual's perception of it and their ability to deal with it.

## How does stress affect the body?

The brain reacts to stress by preparing the body to either stay put and face the perceived threat, or to escape from it. It does this by releasing hormones – chemical messengers – including adrenaline, noradrenaline and cortisol, into the bloodstream. These speed up the heart rate and breathing patterns and may induce sweating. Glucose and fatty acid levels in the blood rise, to provide a burst of energy to deal with the threat by challenging it or running away. This is called the 'fight or flight' response.

Nowadays, the situations that induce this stress response are unlikely to necessitate either of these reactions, but the body continues to respond in the way it has been programmed to do. Stressful situations that continue over a long period of time with no end in sight, for example long-term unemployment, illness or an unhappy relationship, mean that stress hormone levels remain high, thereby increasing the risk of major health problems such as coronary heart disease, as well as other psychological and physical symptoms. These include irritability, poor concentration, anxiety and depression, headaches, skin problems and allergies, such as hay fever.

## How is stress involved in hay fever?

A study at Ohio State University in 2008 involving 28 people suggested that stress makes hay fever symptoms worse. The participants were tested with various substances and their reactions were noted. They were then divided into two groups.

The first group went through a low-stress test that involved reading a magazine article alone and then recording themselves reading it out loud. After the experiment, this group showed no difference in the size of the skin wheal they developed in response to a known allergen.

The second group was asked to do a more stressful test. They each had to deliver a ten-minute speech to a group of 'behavioural experts' and then solve maths problems in their head whilst being videotaped. In this group, the skin wheals they developed after contact with a known allergen were double the size noted in the initial tests. Researchers also reported that this group was more than four times as likely to have a heightened response to the allergen the following day. This suggests that just one stressful event can have a prolonged effect on your immune response.

This study demonstrates the extent to which stress is implicated in hay fever and highlights the important role stress management could play in controlling your symptoms. The stress the second group experienced was the type many of us encounter on a daily basis.

## What can I do about stress?

There are basically three things you can do to manage stress: avoid it, reduce it and relieve it.

## 24. Keep a stress diary

Over a couple of weeks, note down the details of situations, times, places and people that make you feel stressed. Once you've identified these, think about each one and ask yourself: 'Can I avoid it?' For example, if driving to work during the rush hour makes you feel extremely stressed, perhaps you can avoid doing it by starting or finishing work a little earlier or later. If you cannot avoid it, you can usually reduce the level of stress you experience by changing your attitude or by taking practical steps to help you cope better. You can also relieve the effects of stress by practising relaxation techniques and doing things that help you unwind.

### Remember that you'll never reach the end of your 'to-do list'

Workaholism is another factor that tends to be linked with perfectionism – a 'perfect' home and lifestyle have to be paid for.

Whilst working hard for what you want in life is commendable, some people work such long hours that they don't have time to enjoy what they have. If you're constantly driven to get everything done, and think you'll feel calm and relaxed once everything on your 'to-do list' is completed, think again! What tends to happen is that, as you complete tasks, you add new ones to your list, so you never get to the end of it. It's a fact of life that there will always be tasks to be completed. Dr Carlson suggests you remind yourself that, when you die, you will leave behind unfinished business!

## 25. Try not to worry

Worrying about events that haven't even happened can bring on the stress response, as your body can't differentiate between what has actually happened and what you imagine happening. For example, if you are worried about being made redundant or paying your mortgage, your body will produce stress hormones, even if you don't actually lose your job or your home. Although it's hard not to worry about the things that might go wrong in your life, it's better for your health if you can make a conscious decision not to worry about things that haven't happened yet.

### Remind yourself life is OK
As well as recognising the external factors that make you feel stressed, consider whether some aspects of your personality are also to blame. Are you a perfectionist who is never satisfied with your achievements and lifestyle? Constantly feeling that who you are, and what you have, aren't good enough, can lead to unrealistic expectations, discontent and unnecessary pressure. Instead, learn to value your

accomplishments and what you already have. In his best-selling book *Don't Sweat the Small Stuff*, Dr Richard Carlson urges us to remind ourselves that 'life is okay the way it is, right now'. Adopting this attitude immediately reduces stress and induces calm.

## 26. Change your attitude

When difficult situations do come along, changing your attitude towards them can reduce the amount of stress they cause, because it is your interpretation of the event, not the event itself, that elicits your emotional response. When something bad happens, instead of thinking about how awful the situation is, try to find something positive about it if you can. Try to find positive solutions to your problems, or view them as opportunities for personal growth. For example, being made redundant initially seems like a negative event but, if you view it as an opportunity to retrain and start a new career doing something you really enjoy, it can become a catalyst for positive change.

### Live in the moment

Living in the moment, or practising mindfulness, has been shown to reduce stress levels. It involves giving all of your attention to the here and now, rather than worrying about the past or future, and has its roots in Buddhism. It's based on the philosophy that you can't alter the past, or foretell the future, but you can influence what's happening in your life right now. By living fully in the present, you can perform to the best of your ability, whereas worrying about the past and future can hamper how you function now, and increase your stress levels unnecessarily.

Living in this way means your experience of life is richer, because instead of doing things on autopilot, all of your senses will be fully engaged in what you are doing. Imagine going for a walk in the park whilst being so preoccupied with worries about the future, or regrets about the past, that you don't even notice your surroundings. Then think how much more pleasurable and relaxing the experience would be if you took the time to absorb the sights, sounds and smells around you. When you focus on the here and now, you will find yourself appreciating the simple things in your life more.

Mindfulness is also about being happy with your life as it is now, rather than thinking you can only be happy when you've achieved certain things, such as a better job, a bigger house, etc. Octavius Black, co-author of *The Mind Gym: Give Me Time*, suggests that we should 'make today be tomorrow's happy memories'. Adopting this attitude towards life will immediately lower your stress levels. If you find it hard to focus on the present, try keeping a daily diary.

## 27. Simplify your life

If you feel that your life is spiralling out of control with too many demands from work, your home, your partner, your family and friends, maybe it's time to simplify your life. If you regularly feel under pressure and stressed because of a lack of time, try reviewing how you use it. Keep a diary for a few days to see how you spend your time and then decide which activities you can cut out or reduce to make more time for the things that are most important to you. Try saying 'no' to the non-essential tasks you don't have time for, or just don't want to do. It's a little word, but it can dramatically reduce your stress levels. If you find it hard to say no, then perhaps you need to develop your assertiveness skills.

## Slow down

Many of us are living our lives at a faster and faster pace, perhaps juggling a full-time job with a relationship, family commitments and a social life. As a result, we feel a constant sense of urgency in our daily lives as we race from one task to another. This constant feeling of pressure fuels our impatience when we have to wait in a queue or a traffic jam, or if the bus or train is late. Octavius Black says we need to accept that we will never have enough time to do everything. He believes that, in order to enjoy the moment, we need to slow down, perhaps viewing situations such as queuing or travel delays as welcome thinking or reading time, rather than allowing impatience and frustration to raise our stress levels unnecessarily.

### Prioritise

When you have a long 'to-do' list, number tasks in terms of urgency and importance and carry them out in that order.

## Delegate

Perfectionism can also lead to a need to control – you convince yourself that no one else can meet your high standards, so you do everything yourself. This inevitably leads to physical and mental overload. The solution is to accept that you can't know and do everything, so you need to learn to listen to other people's ideas and opinions and to delegate. Ask your partner and children to help with domestic tasks. Accept any offers of help at work.

### Clear away clutter

If a bulging wardrobe, heaving shelves and overflowing cupboards are getting you down, make your life simpler and less stressful by getting rid of unnecessary clutter around your home. You'll save time, because you'll find things more quickly in a clutter-free environment, and your mental clarity will improve, because ridding yourself of physical clutter clears mental clutter. If you haven't worn, read, or used an item for two years or more, give it to a charity shop, sell it on eBay, or bin it. If you can't bear to get rid of it, store it in the loft – then make it a rule that if you haven't thought about using the item within six months, it is time to part with it. If you have a lot of possessions to sort out, ask your partner, a family member or a friend to help you. You'll be amazed at how much happier and less stressed you will feel after a good clear out.

## 28. Assert yourself

If you feel you often hide your true feelings instead of expressing them, and give in to others so that you don't hurt or upset them or to gain their approval, you might benefit from brushing up your assertiveness skills.

Do you regularly allow others to manipulate you into doing things you don't want to do? Being assertive empowers you to say what you want, feel and need, calmly and confidently, without being aggressive or hurting others. Try the following techniques to develop your self-assertiveness, so that you remain in control of your life and do things because *you* want to, rather than to please other people.

☐ Demonstrate ownership of your thoughts, feelings and behaviour by using 'I' rather than 'we', 'you' or 'it'. Rather than saying 'You make me angry', try something like 'I feel angry when you...'. This is less antagonising to the other person.

☐ When you have a choice whether to do something or not, say 'won't' rather than 'can't' to show that you've made an active decision, rather than suggesting that something or someone has stopped you. Say 'choose to' instead of 'have to' and 'could' rather than 'should', to indicate that you have a choice. For example: 'I won't be going out tonight', rather than 'I can't go out tonight', or 'I could go out tonight, but I have chosen to stay in.'

☐ When you feel that your needs aren't being considered, state what you want calmly and clearly, repeating it until the other person shows they've heard and understood what you've said.

☐ When making a request, identify exactly what it is you want and what you're prepared to settle for. Choose positive, assertive words, as outlined above. For example: 'I would like you to help me tidy the kitchen. I'd really appreciate it if you could empty the kitchen bin.'

☐ When refusing a request, speak calmly but firmly, giving the reason or reasons why, without apologising. Repeat if you need to. For example: 'I won't be able to babysit for you tonight because I'm feeling really tired after being at work all day.'

When you disagree with someone, say so using the word 'I'. Explain why you disagree, but acknowledge the other person's right to have a different viewpoint. For example: 'I don't agree that the service in that restaurant is poor – our meal was only late last time we visited because it was extremely busy, but I can understand why you think that.'

## 29. Seek support

Hay fever can be an isolating and distressing condition with many sufferers feeling that no one understands what they are experiencing. In a recent survey for Kleenex by Professor Jean Emberlin, Director of NPARU, which involved 928 hay fever sufferers, almost two-thirds of those aged 16–24 and over half of those aged 25–34 said that hay fever affected their social lives. Over one in four said it affected their family lives. Making contact with fellow sufferers who are dealing with the same symptoms as you may help you to overcome these feelings. The organisations listed below offer the opportunity to do just that; further information and contact details are listed in the Directory at the end of the book.

**Action Against Allergy** is a UK charity set up to advance understanding and recognition of allergic medical conditions and allergy-related illness. Once you have become a member, you can access Talk Line, the charity's telephone network that enables you to speak to other members who have experienced allergies and can empathise with you.

**Allergy UK** is a leading medical charity dealing with allergies. The charity's website hosts community allergy discussion boards on a variety of topics, including respiratory allergy, which covers hay fever. There is also a helpline.

**Health Boards** offers online community message boards on a variety of health conditions, including allergies.

**Talk Allergy** is a UK website set up by hay fever sufferer Deborah Mason. Once you have registered as a member you can access the message board, which enables you to read and post messages to other hay fever sufferers. You can also use the Find a Friend Pen Pal area and receive an electronic newsletter called *Intouch*.

### Help is at hand

If you feel you can't deal with life's stresses on your own, don't be afraid to seek professional help. Your first port of call should be your doctor, as he or she should be able to offer advice, and possibly refer you to a counsellor.

The Stress Management Society offers further guidance on dealing with stress, including 'desk yoga' and 'desk massage' techniques you can practise at work, and a creative visualisation you can do whenever you have a few minutes to yourself. See the Directory at the end of the book for contact details.

## 30. Sleep soundly

Lack of sleep can increase stress levels, which in turn exacerbates hay fever symptoms. A blocked nose or the pain of sinusitis can disrupt sleep, leading to a continuing cycle of poor sleep patterns, feeling stressed and worsening symptoms.

To sleep more soundly, try the following:

Get outdoors during the day (see Action 6 – Reduce your exposure to pollen/spores). Exposure to daylight stops the production of melatonin, the brain chemical that promotes sleep, making it easier for your body to release it at night so that you fall asleep more easily and sleep more soundly.

Choose foods rich in tryptophan, an amino acid your body uses to produce serotonin (a brain chemical that's converted into the 'sleep hormone' melatonin). Tryptophan-rich foods include bananas, dates, dairy foods, chicken, turkey, rice, oats, wholegrain breads and cereals. Make sure you're neither too hungry nor too full when you go to bed, as both can cause wakefulness.

Don't drink coffee or cola after 2 p.m., because the stimulant effects of the caffeine they contain can last for hours. Whilst tea contains about half as much caffeine – around 50 mg per cup – it's best not to drink it near bedtime if you have difficulty sleeping. Redbush or herb teas, which are caffeine-free, make good alternatives.

Exercise can help you sleep more soundly, because it encourages your body temperature and metabolism to increase and then fall a few hours later, which promotes sleep. Try not to exercise later than early evening, as exercising too late at night can have the opposite effect because the body temperature may still be raised at bedtime. Not taking enough exercise can cause sleep problems and restlessness.

Wind down before bedtime. Develop a regular routine in the evening that allows you to 'put the day to bed'. This could involve watching TV if you find that relaxing, although it's probably best to avoid watching anything that could prey on your mind later on when you are trying to go to sleep. Other relaxing activities you could do include reading, listening to music and having a long soak in a warm bath.

Soak in a warm bath at bedtime. Your temperature increases slightly with the warmth and then falls – helping you to drop off. Add a few drops of essential oils such as lavender or chamomile for their soothing properties.

Avoid drinking alcohol at bedtime: although it may relax you at first and help you fall asleep more quickly, it has a stimulant effect, causing you to awaken more often during the night. It's also a diuretic, making nocturnal trips to the toilet more likely. But, if abstinence doesn't help you sleep better, it may be worth indulging in a glass of Cabernet Sauvignon, Merlot or Chianti at bedtime – there's some evidence that these wines improve your sleep patterns, because the grape skins they contain are rich in plant melatonin.

○ Ensure your bedroom is cool and dark. Your brain tries to reduce your body temperature at night to slow down your metabolism. So to encourage sleep, aim for a temperature of around 16°C. Darkness stimulates the pineal gland in the brain to produce melatonin.

○ To help your brain associate the bedroom with sleep and sex only, avoid having a TV or computer in your bedroom. Watching TV or using a computer last thing at night can overstimulate your brain, making it harder for you to switch off and fall asleep. Also, both TV and computer screens emit bright light that may interfere with the production of melatonin.

○ Only go to bed when you feel really sleepy. If you can't drop off within what seems like around 20 minutes, get up and do something you find relaxing but not too stimulating, such as reading or listening to calming music. Only return to your bed when you feel sleepy again – this helps to reinforce your brain's connection between your bed and sleep.

○ If mulling over problems or a busy schedule the next day stops you from falling asleep, try writing down your concerns or a plan for the day ahead before you go to bed.

### Sprinkle eucalyptus oil

If a blocked nose prevents sleep, try sprinkling 2–3 drops of eucalyptus oil on your pillow at night.

## 31. Laugh more

Laughter is a great stress reliever. A good belly laugh seems to reduce the stress hormones cortisol and adrenaline and raise mood-boosting serotonin levels. People who see the funny side of life appear to have a reduced risk of the health problems associated with stress, including hay fever and other allergies. Researchers at the American College of Cardiology recently reported that 15 minutes of laughter a day can reduce allergy symptoms by boosting chemicals that block the release of histamine. So make time to watch your favourite comedies and comedians and be around people who make you laugh. Or visit www.laughlab.co.uk or www.ahajokes.com whenever you feel like a good giggle!

## 32. Do something purely for pleasure

Spend time each day doing something purely for pleasure – whether it's luxuriating in a warm, scented bath with a glass of wine and a good book, listening to your favourite music, or going to the cinema. Doing something you really enjoy will help to take your mind off domestic and work pressures.

**Pucker up**

Scientists in Japan recently reported that kissing suppresses the body's allergic reaction to pollen by relaxing the body and reducing the amount of histamine produced.

## 33. Get the exercise habit

Regular exercise is a great antidote to stress, because it enables the body to utilise the stress hormones whose purpose is to provide the extra energy needed to run away from our aggressors, or to stay put and fight. It also triggers the release of endorphins, which act as natural painkillers and antidepressants.

Swimming is a good all-round exercise and many people find being in the water relaxing. For information about swimming lessons, visit www.swimtime.org and to improve your swimming technique from your desk, visit www.swimfit.com, a website that offers animated swimming stroke guides. Tai Chi, described as a 'moving meditation', may also help to reduce stress whilst helping you to keep fit – for classes near you visit www.taichifinder.co.uk.

However, you don't need to join a class to become more active: incorporating exercise into your daily routine is easy and just as effective. Putting more effort into the housework, gardening, walking the dog, getting up from your desk and walking around regularly, and walking whilst talking on a mobile are all ways of being more active. When pollen/spore levels are very high, either exercise indoors or follow the strategies aimed at reducing your exposure – see Chapter 3.

## 34. Consider ecotherapy

Researchers at Essex University say that ecotherapy (engaging with nature) offers both mental and physical health benefits. Whether through an active pursuit such as walking or gardening, or a passive one like admiring the view, being close to nature has been shown to reduce stress and ease muscular tension. Experts claim that the higher levels of negative ions near areas with running water, trees and mountains may play a part. Others suggest that the success of ecotherapy is down to 'biophilia' – the theory that we all have an innate affinity with nature and that our 'disconnection' from it is the cause of stress and mental health problems. Studies in the Netherlands and Japan suggest that people living in or near green areas enjoy a longer and healthier life than those living in urban environments. Whilst engaging with nature is more difficult for hay fever sufferers – especially during the height of the pollen or season – it isn't impossible. Follow the advice on reducing your exposure to pollen and other allergens in Chapter 3.

## 35. Practise muscle relaxation

This technique, known as Progressive Muscle Relaxation, helps to release tension from the muscles. According to Richard Hilliard, director of the Relaxation for Living Institute (RFL), it's impossible to have an anxious mind when your muscles are relaxed. The Institute's website offers advice on relaxation and stress management.

Try following these steps whenever you feel tense and anxious. Alternatively you can buy a guided deep relaxation as an MP3 download on the RFL website (see Directory).

Take a deep breath and then create tension in your face by clenching your teeth and screwing up your eyes tightly, then relax and breathe out.

Take a deep breath, then lift the muscles in your shoulders, tense them for a few seconds and then relax, dropping your shoulders and releasing the tension as you breathe out.

Take a deep breath, then clench your fists and tense the muscles in your arms, hold for a few seconds then release and breathe out.

Next, tense the muscles in your buttocks and both of your legs, including the thighs and calves, hold, and then release as you breathe out.

Finally, clench your toes and tense your feet, hold, and then release and breathe out.

## 36. Meditate

Research suggests that meditation lowers stress. There are various meditation techniques, but here is a simple one that can be practised whenever you have a few moments to yourself – even whilst on the bus or train!

Close your eyes and focus on your breathing. As you inhale slowly and deeply through your nose, expand your stomach, hold for a few seconds, before drawing in your stomach, whilst exhaling slowly. Whenever your attention is distracted by a passing thought, return to simply observing your breathing. If you prefer, you can listen to a step-by-step mindfulness meditation at www.stressmanagement.co.uk.

### Try complementary therapies

Various complementary therapies, including acupressure, aromatherapy, massage, reflexology and yoga, are thought to help relieve psychological stress and muscle tension. For ideas on how you can practise these therapies at home, see Chapter 8 – DIY Complementary Therapies.

**Chapter 6**

# Medical Treatments

As we have discussed in the previous chapters, your best defences against hay fever are avoiding your allergens, managing stress and eating a balanced diet. If you do all you can to prevent hay fever symptoms developing in the first place, you will need less medication and will suffer fewer side effects and interactions. However, although you may experience a reduction in the frequency and severity of your symptoms, there are no miracle cures for hay fever, so it is likely that, at times, you will still need to resort to medications to prevent and treat it. If you know the time of year you usually develop hay fever, you should begin treatment before the symptoms set in, because they are more difficult to treat once they are fully established. Sometimes a combination of treatments is more beneficial, and you may need to try several different medications before you find those that suit you best.

This chapter gives an overview of the over-the-counter and prescription-only medications commonly used to treat hay fever, such as antihistamines, decongestants, sodium cromoglicate, ipratropium bromide, corticosteroids and immunotherapy, including what they are, how they work and possible side effects. Details of a relatively new treatment for hay fever, called phototherapy, are also given. Not everyone will suffer side effects from taking medications, and there may be others in addition to those listed – always read the leaflet that accompanies the medication and discuss any concerns with your pharmacist or GP before using it. Always inform your GP or pharmacist if you are taking any vitamin, mineral or herbal supplements, as these may interact with medications, or reduce their effectiveness.

### Money-saving tip

Ask your pharmacist for generic versions of these medications. They are the same drugs, but without the brand name, and can be up to 75 per cent cheaper.

## 37. Learn about medications for hay fever

### Antihistamines

Antihistamines relieve hay fever symptoms by blocking the release of histamine in the body. They are available in tablet, spray, or syrup form. Nasal sprays act quickly and can start to ease an itchy, runny nose and sneezing within 15 minutes. Newer or 'second-generation' antihistamines cause less drowsiness than the older ones, such as chlorphenamine (Piriton), although some people may still be affected by them – especially if they are combined with alcohol.

The newer antihistamines include acrivastine, cetirizine, desloratidine, fexofenadine and loratadine.

## Acrivastine

Acrivastine is a non-sedating antihistamine that doesn't usually cause any severe side effects, but some people still experience drowsiness and blurred vision, so check that your reaction times are normal before operating machinery or driving. Drink alcohol in moderation, as it will make any drowsiness worse. Acrivastine may cause a dry mouth – chewing sugar-free gum may help. Other possible side effects include headache, tummy upset, dizziness and disturbed sleep. This medication can also increase sensitivity to sunlight. Over-the-counter medications containing acrivastine include Benadryl Allergy Relief and Benadryl Plus, which also contains the decongestant pseudoephedrine. Both are in capsule form.

## Cetirizine

Cetirizine is usually well tolerated, but it still can cause drowsiness in some people. If you are affected, you shouldn't drive or operate machinery. It may also cause a dry mouth, headache, blurred vision and tummy upsets. You shouldn't take cetirizine during pregnancy or whilst breastfeeding. Well-known over-the-counter brands that contain cetirizine include Zirtek, Benadryl One-a-Day Relief and Galpharm Hayfever and Allergy Relief One-a-Day Tablets. Cetirizine is also available on prescription as tablets and as an oral solution for children.

## Desloratidine

Less than one in ten people might experience tiredness, drowsiness, a dry mouth or headaches whilst taking this medication. Very rare side effects include tummy upsets and sleep problems. Inform your GP or pharmacist if you are pregnant, trying for a baby or breastfeeding, or if you have kidney problems, epilepsy, porphyria (a metabolic abnormality), or an intolerance to some sugars. It is available as a prescription-only medicine called NeoClarityn as tablets and as an oral solution.

## Fexofenadine

Possible but rare side effects from using fexofenadine include headache, blurred vision, drowsiness, dry mouth and increased sensitivity to sunlight. Let your GP or pharmacist know if you are pregnant, trying for a baby or breastfeeding, or if you suffer from heart problems, epilepsy or porphyria before taking fexofenadine. This antihistamine is available as prescription-only tablets under the brand name Telfast for those aged 12 and over.

## Loratadine

This is another non-drowsy antihistamine – though it can cause drowsiness in some users. Other possible side effects include blurred vision and a dry mouth. Loratadine isn't recommended during pregnancy or whilst breastfeeding. If you are pregnant or breastfeeding, or suffer from kidney or liver problems, epilepsy or porphyria, let your GP or pharmacist know before taking it. It is available over the counter as Clarityn Allergy Tablets and Clarityn Allergy Syrup (fast acting and suitable for adults as well as children aged 2–12 years) and on prescription, as an oral solution for children and as tablets for people aged 12 and over.

# Antihistamine nasal sprays and eye drops

Antihistamines available as nasal sprays and eye drops include azelastine and antazoline.

## Azelastine: nasal spray

Azelastine works better than oral antihistamines for hay fever symptoms affecting the nose, but doesn't help with those affecting the eyes. Because it is sprayed into the nose, it acts directly on the membranes, blocking the effects of histamines and preventing the release of other allergy chemicals. It acts more quickly than tablets and is unlikely to cause drowsiness. It can be used both to prevent and relieve the nasal symptoms of hay fever. Possible side effects include nausea and a bitter taste in the mouth, nasal irritation, sneezing and nose bleeds. The safety of using this medication during pregnancy hasn't been determined yet – it may pass into breast milk, so seek advice from your GP first. It is available as a prescription-only medication called Rhinolast and is suitable for use from the age of five years.

### Nasal spray tip

When using an azelastine nasal spray, hold your head upright to prevent the medication from trickling down the back of your throat and causing a bitter taste in the mouth.

### Azelastine: eye drops

Azelastine eye drops relieve the eye symptoms of hay fever by blocking the effects of histamine. They are effective in about 50 per cent of users. Azelastine eye drops aren't recommended for children under the age of four. If you are pregnant, attempting to become pregnant or breastfeeding, inform your GP or pharmacist before using this medication.

### Antazoline eye drops

Antazoline is available in over-the-counter eye drops under the brand name Otrivine antistin, which also contain the decongestant xylometazoline (see below). Antazoline blocks the effects of histamine, while xylometazoline constricts the blood vessels in the eyes, reducing the amount of histamine reaching the eye membranes and relieving redness. These eye drops aren't suitable for soft contact lens wearers. They may cause temporary blurring of vision – you are advised not to drive or operate machinery until these effects have worn off. The drops shouldn't be used for more than seven consecutive days without seeing your GP, pharmacist or optician. Always see your GP if your symptoms don't improve within two days of using these drops, as this may mean you have an eye infection.

## Decongestants

Decongestants clear a blocked nose, enabling you to breathe more easily. They work by constricting the blood vessels in the nose, which reduces the swelling and cuts the production of mucus. They don't affect the release of antihistamine and other chemicals involved in the allergic response. Their use should be limited to seven consecutive days, as they can cause 'rebound' congestion if they are used over a longer period of time, and increased doses may be needed to achieve the same results. Constant long-term use could lead to chronic sinusitis and damage the nasal passages, which can reduce the sense of smell. These are available in nasal spray, tablet and liquid form. Commonly used decongestants include oxymetazoline, xylometazoline and pseudoephedrine.

### Oxymetazoline
Possible side effects of oxymetazoline include nasal irritation, sneezing, dry mouth and throat and rebound congestion when used over a prolonged period of time. This medication should be used with caution if you suffer from coronary heart disease, high blood pressure, an overactive thyroid, diabetes mellitus, glaucoma or an enlarged prostate gland. If you are pregnant or breastfeeding you should seek medical advice before using medications containing

oxymetazoline. Children under six years of age should not use this medicine. Also, anyone who has taken monoamine-oxidase inhibitor (MAOI) antidepressants should not use this medication within two weeks of taking them because the combined effects could cause dangerously high blood pressure. Well-known brands containing oxymetazoline include Vicks Sinex Decongestant Nasal Spray, Nasivin Decongestant Nasal Spray and Afrazine Nasal Spray.

## Xylometazoline

Possible side effects of this medication include nasal irritation, burning, stinging or dryness, sneezing, headaches and nausea. This medicine should be used with caution if you suffer from heart disease, high blood pressure, diabetes or an overactive thyroid. It should not be used during pregnancy and you should seek medical advice before using it whilst breastfeeding. It shouldn't be used by anyone who has taken MAOI antidepressants in the previous two weeks, or by anyone who has had neurosurgery or had their pituitary gland surgically removed. Well-known brands containing xylometazoline include Otrivine Adult Menthol Nasal Spray, Otrivine Child Nasal Drops and Sudafed Decongestant Nasal Spray.

## Pseudoephedrine

Possible side effects include a dry mouth, nose or throat, anxiety, restlessness, disturbed sleep, increased heart rate, a skin rash, difficulty in passing urine, and hallucinations. Pseudoephedrine should be used with caution if you have decreased kidney or liver function, heart disease, high blood pressure, diabetes, an overactive thyroid, an enlarged prostate gland, or glaucoma. Children under the age of 12 shouldn't use this medication. If you are pregnant or breastfeeding, you should seek medical advice before using this medicine. Don't take this medicine if you have very high blood pressure (hypertension), severe coronary heart disease or have taken MAOI antidepressants in the previous 14 days. Well-known over-the-counter products containing pseudoephedrine include Sudafed 12-Hour Relief Tablets and Sudafed Children's Syrup. Prescription-only drugs containing pseudoephedrine include Galpseud non-drowsy tablets and linctus and Contac non-drowsy 12-hour relief capsules.

## Other treatments

### Sodium cromoglicate: nasal spray

Sodium cromoglicate is an anti-inflammatory drug. It is thought to work by 'stabilising' mast cells and preventing the release of histamine. It is available as a nasal spray and eye drops.

Sodium cromoglicate nasal spray provides relief from a blocked or runny nose, sneezing and itching. GPs often recommend it for children, if your symptoms are mild, or if you are already taking prescribed steroids for another condition. It is recommended that you start using it at least a week before you expect your symptoms to start and that you use it regularly, even when you don't have symptoms, to prevent them developing. Sodium cromoglicate nasal spray is available over the counter at pharmacies as Resiston 1 or Vividrin Nasal Spray and on prescription as Rynacrom. Occasionally, there may be nasal irritation during the first few days of use. Other reported but rare side effects include wheezing or chest tightness. Caution is advised during pregnancy, especially in the first trimester, but it is thought to be safe for use during breastfeeding

### Sodium cromoglicate: eye drops

Sodium cromoglicate is also available over the counter as eye drops to both prevent and relieve eye symptoms like itchiness and grittiness. These eye drops can't be used whilst wearing contact lenses. Possible side effects include temporary stinging, burning, or blurred vision. As with the nasal spray, caution is advised during pregnancy, especially in the first trimester, but it is thought to be safe for use during breastfeeding. Over-the-counter eye drops containing sodium cromoglicate include Clarityn Allergy, Opticrom Allergy, Optrex Allergy Eyes, Galpharm Allergy Eye Drops, Pollenase Allergy Eye Drops and Vividrin Hay Fever. Prescription-only medications include Hay Crom Eye Drops, Vividrin and Opticrom Eye drops.

## Treatments for persistent symptoms

### Ipratropium bromide: nasal spray

Ipratropium bromide belongs to a group of medicines called antimuscarinics. It is effective at relieving a persistently runny nose because it reduces the amount of mucus produced. It works by blocking the actions of a natural chemical called acetycholine, which is involved in the production of mucus. Possible side effects include a dry, sore, itchy nose and blood in your mucus. Rarer side effects include a sore throat, headaches and nausea. If you are pregnant or breastfeeding, or suffer from cystic fibrosis, glaucoma, or an enlarged prostate gland, inform your GP or pharmacist before using this medication. Ipratropium bromide is prescription-only (brand name Rinatec).

### Corticosteroids

Corticosteroids, otherwise known as steroids, have powerful anti-inflammatory effects and are mainly used in nasal spray or tablet form. Steroid injections were used to treat hay fever in the past, but they're not used very often now because of the risk of severe side effects. Taking steroids orally can also cause serious side effects, such as osteoporosis, reduced immunity, stomach ulcers and high blood pressure, so doctors usually initially prescribe corticosteroid nasal sprays, as the risks are lower.

## Corticosteroids: nasal sprays

Corticosteroid nasal sprays often relieve persistent nasal symptoms such as a blocked or runny nose better than antihistamine tablets and may also improve eye symptoms. To get the maximum benefit from nasal corticosteroids sprays, you need to start using them a couple of weeks before you expect your symptoms to start and then to use them regularly. Over-the-counter steroid nasal sprays include Beconase and Flixonase. Other preparations are available on prescription, such as budesonide, which is also known as Rhinocort Aqua. Some people find that steroid sprays cause mild irritation and nosebleeds. Although the risks are lower than those associated with taking steroids in tablet form, high doses used over a prolonged period may lead to the development of the more serious side effects linked to corticosteroids – so always use the lowest dose that works for you. Because of these risks, children can only use a steroid spray when it is prescribed; alternatively, another type of nasal spray containing sodium cromoglicate, called Rynacrom, might be suggested (see above).

## Corticosteroids: tablets

Corticosteroid tablets (brand name Prednisolone) are sometimes prescribed for hay fever, but only as a last resort to provide relief from severe symptoms when other forms of prevention and treatment have failed to work, and they should only be used for a short period of time.

# Immunotherapy

Your GP or allergy specialist may prescribe immunotherapy if other preventative and symptom-relief treatments have proved ineffective. Immunotherapy works by exposing your body to tiny amounts of modified forms of your particular allergens in order to gradually desensitise your body, so that it no longer produces histamine and other allergy chemicals when it encounters them. There are two types of immunotherapy – one is delivered by injection, under the brand name Pollinex Quattro, and the other through sub-lingual tablets (tablets which dissolve under the tongue) with the brand name Grazax.

## Pollinex Quattro

The Pollinex Quattro treatment programme consists of just four injections and should be started two to four months before the pollen season starts. It carries a small risk of provoking a severe reaction (anaphylaxis), so it is usually carried out at specialist allergy centres. It aims to reduce allergies to various grasses, rye, and alder, birch and hazel tree pollens. Clinical trials reported statistically significant improvements in the symptoms and quality of life of those who took part.

## Grazax

Grazax tablets contain an extract of timothy grass pollen and should be taken once a day – ideally starting a minimum of four months before the pollen season begins. Clinical trials reported a reduction in symptoms and a 40–60 per cent reduction in the need for medication. There were only minor side effects, such as itchiness in the mouth and mild swelling. Although there were no severe allergic reactions during the trial, it is recommended that the first dose is given at a clinic. After that, the tablets can be taken at home. For the best results, Grazax should be viewed as a fairly long-term treatment and taken for up to three years – though there is usually an improvement in symptoms after a few months. It is only effective for people who are allergic to timothy grass pollen.

## Phototherapy

Phototherapy, also known as light therapy, was developed in hospitals for treating allergic conditions like eczema. It uses UV light to stop the release of histamine, which reduces allergic symptoms such as congestion, runny nose, watery eyes and headaches. In 2009, a UK study reported that phototherapy was better than a placebo for reducing nasal allergic symptoms such as itching, sneezing and a runny nose, as well as runny eyes and an itchy mouth/palate. The researchers suggested that phototherapy might open up new opportunities for the treatment of hay fever.

## 38. Visit your GP

Your GP or pharmacist will be able to provide you with further details of the medications mentioned above and other treatments for hay fever.

It is a good idea to try to deal with your hay fever symptoms yourself before seeking medical advice. You may find that following the advice in this book (identifying and avoiding your allergens, eating healthily, taking appropriate natural supplements or over-the-counter medications and managing stress) can reduce the frequency and severity of your attacks and may even prevent them. However, if, despite your best efforts, you are still suffering, or you develop a wheeze, it's advisable that you visit your GP. Take along details of when and where your symptoms occur, as this will help your GP to ascertain the likely causes. Your GP may recommend allergy tests to identify the exact cause/s of your hay fever and prescribe more potent medications.

**Chapter 7**

# Living and Working with Hay Fever

Having hay fever can affect your quality of life and research has shown that hay fever symptoms have a negative effect on the academic performance of young children and teenagers. This chapter offers advice on living with hay fever; it includes tips on how to cope whilst at work and at school, how to time holidays to avoid pollen seasons – both at home and abroad – and how to minimise the effects that hay fever has on your appearance.

## Coping with hay fever at work

According to recent research by Professor Emberlin (see Chapter 5 – Hay Fever and Emotions), almost 40 per cent of hay fever sufferers admitted that they struggled to concentrate at work during an attack. Over a third believed their productivity was up to a quarter lower when their symptoms were at their worst.

However, the 401 managers surveyed revealed that they didn't notice this reduction in productivity and less than half offered any help (e.g. tissues or air filters) to ease the symptoms of employees with hay fever. Most said they wouldn't allow staff to stay at home when the pollen count was high and a quarter would question an employee's commitment to their job if they called in sick because of hay fever. This explains why nearly eight out of ten hay fever sufferers surveyed said they wouldn't take time off work due to severe hay fever symptoms. Fewer than two people out of ten said they would admit to being absent from work because of hay fever.

## 39. Reduce symptoms at work

The best way to stop hay fever from impacting on your working life is to aim to prevent your symptoms as much as possible. Following the advice in this book regarding monitoring the pollen count, taking appropriate medications and modifying your diet and lifestyle will go a long way to help. Other things you could do include:

- Keep a supply of any medication or supplements you use to control your symptoms at work in your desk drawer.

- Carry a 'hay fever kit'– this could consist of tissues and a pot of vaseline to trap pollen and protect the skin around your nose.

- Take some cleaning wipes to work so that you can wipe down your desk and chair to remove pollen.

- If your office doesn't have air conditioning, ask your employer to consider installing it, or take a personal air filter to work with you (see the Useful Products section).

### Talk to your employer

Although some bosses appear to be unsympathetic towards hay fever sufferers, it's still a good idea to make sure that your boss is aware of the impact your symptoms have on you. If you feel too unwell, or are too embarassed by your appearance to face going in to work, you could offer to complete some work from home – although this may be met with a lack of enthusiasm, it at least shows a commitment to your job. However, if, despite following prevention strategies and using appropriate medications, your symptoms are so severe you are unable to work, you should consider visiting your GP, who might suggest other, more effective treatments.

## Living with hay fever: children

About a third of people who have hay fever develop it during childhood, usually between the ages of five and ten. Older children and teenagers are more likely to suffer from hay fever than adults. Hay fever can be particularly difficult for children to cope with, as they may be too young to understand why they are suffering. A stuffy nose and itchy eyes might make sleep difficult and even affect the appetite.

## 40. Help your child to cope with hay fever at school

Hay fever symptoms can be especially difficult to handle during school hours, when children have to concentrate and don't have a parent around to help them deal with their symptoms. Make sure your child takes their medication before going to school, as most schools stipulate that the parent or guardian should administer medicines. The exception is if your child uses an inhaler – schools usually allow access to these at all times. Ensuring your child takes appropriate hay fever medications will mean that he or she can enjoy the health and social benefits of outdoor playtime without making their symptoms worse.

### Talk to your child's teacher

If your child suffers from hay fever, it's important that you make their teacher aware of it, so that they offer your child support and understanding – especially if he or she is feeling tired and miserable, or unable to concentrate. The teacher may even offer to discuss allergies during PSHE (Personal, Health and Social Education) lessons, so that other children are more understanding.

Unfortunately, exam time tends to coincide with the period when the grass pollen season is at its peak and hay fever prevalence is at its highest. Research suggests that up to 40 per cent of pupils who suffer from hay fever on the day of an exam can drop at least one grade. This is largely due to their symptoms and resulting lack of sleep, as well as the sedative effects of some hay fever medications, affecting their ability to concentrate. If you think your child's performance is affected by his or her symptoms or medication, it's important to let the teacher know. Make sure your child is taking one of the newer antihistamines that are less likely to have a sedative effect, such as acrivastine, cetirizine, desloratidine, fexofenadine or loratadine (see Chapter 6). If your child does suffer from hay fever on the day of an exam, make sure he or she applies for 'special consideration' which, if accepted, could mean being awarded up to two per cent more marks.

## 41. Make a 'hay fever kit' for your child

To help your child cope with hay fever at school, make sure they have a 'hay fever kit', which could consist of one or two packets of tissues, a small pot of vaseline to use as a pollen barrier and also to protect the skin around the nose from constant rubbing, and an inhaler, if he or she is prescribed one.

## 42. Instil confidence in your child

A child with hay fever may be embarrassed by their symptoms and feel isolated from children who don't have the condition. As well as making sure your child takes appropriate medication, carries a 'hay fever kit', and that his or her teacher is informed, it's important to acknowledge his or her discomfort and offer praise for the way he or she is dealing with the symptoms. Explain how common hay fever is – especially if your child doesn't know anyone else with the condition.

## 43. Manage your hay fever on holiday

Most people's main holiday will tend to coincide with the pollen season, both in the UK and abroad. However, it is possible to time your holidays to avoid the pollen season as much as possible.

In the UK, avoid 'hay fever hotspots' – cities with high levels of pollen and pollution and inland lowland areas like the Midlands where pollen counts can be high, and head for the coast, as sea breezes disperse pollen. Mountainous areas like the Scottish Highlands, the Peak District in Derbyshire and Snowdonia in Wales, and moors such as those found in Devon, Cornwall and Yorkshire, are lower-risk areas because the vegetation tends to be allergen-free.

### Pollen seasons abroad

If you are planning to holiday abroad, remember that the pollen seasons vary in different countries. Below is an overview:

### Spain, southern Italy, southern Greece and the Balearics
In these parts of the Mediterranean, the grass pollen season is shorter than that of the UK, running from April until early July. All types of pollen are at their lowest levels from late July to December, making this a good time to holiday in these countries.

## Mediterranean islands

Mediterranean islands, such as Cyprus and Malta, have especially low pollen counts because of sparse vegetation and sea breezes.

## France

In France, the grass pollen season is shorter than in the UK, running from May until early August. However, the tree pollen season is longer, running from January until August, and the weed pollen season runs from March to April and June to September. Remember that coastal and mountainous areas tend to have lower pollen counts.

## Austria, Germany, Scandinavia and Switzerland

If you are allergic to birch pollen and thinking of visiting Austria, Germany, Scandinavia or Switzerland, bear in mind that levels in these countries can be extremely high.

## Tropical areas

Tropical areas tend to have airborne pollen all year round, but you can avoid the peak times. For example, if you are allergic to grass pollen, avoid visiting the Carribean from October to March, or June to July when grass pollen levels peak. Avoid going to Florida between April and October. From January to May, tree pollen levels are high there, as are weed pollen concentrations during May to November.

The website www.nasalairguard.com offers a useful international pollen calendar covering some of these and other countries. Remember that pollen seasons can vary abroad, just as they can in the UK, so if your holiday is likely to be close to one, make sure you go prepared, as it may be difficult for you to obtain your usual medication there. Many countries now provide local pollen information. A website you may find useful when planning a holiday is http://uk.weather.com, which provides pollen counts for major cities around the world.

## 44. Improve your appearance

The Kleenex study reported that, during an attack, a quarter of hay fever sufferers said they were so embarrassed by their appearance that their social life suffered. Over half said they felt less attractive during the peak of the pollen season. I know from my own experience that pink, swollen eyes, a red nose and peeling skin is not a good look!

Trying to improve your appearance with make-up could make sore skin and eyes worse, as cosmetics often contain sensitisers (substances that can provoke an allergic reaction), such as lanolin, fragrance, dyes and preservatives, like parabens, and hay fever is often associated with sensitive skin. However, you should find that your skin and eyes can tolerate hypoallergenic make-up by companies like Almay and Clinique. Mineral make-up, made from crushed minerals such as titanium dioxide and zinc oxide, is said to be less irritating to sensitive skin than conventional make-up. It is also claimed to present virtually no allergy risk and to have a soothing, calming, anti-inflammatory effect on the skin, making it ideal during a hay fever attack. Titanium dioxide is a natural sunscreen, whilst zinc oxide helps to heal the skin. Iredale Mineral Makeup and Lily Lolo Mineral Cosmetics offer a wide range of mineral make-up products: for further details, see the Useful Products section. Mineral make-up is also available from high street make-up brands like Maybelline and Max Factor.

It's probably best to avoid wearing mascara, as it traps pollen – you could try having your eyelashes dyed instead. However, if you prefer to use mascara, choose a waterproof one that won't run when your eyes are streaming. Waterproof mascara is also less likely to flake and get into your eyes, which could cause even more irritation. Make sure it's hypoallergenic too – again, one from the Almay and Clinique range would probably be suitable. It's a good idea to avoid using face powder or powder blusher, as particles may get into your eyes, and go for cream eyeshadows rather than powder ones, as these may also get into your eyes.

It's essential that you remove all make-up, including eye make-up, at night, to give your skin a chance to recover. Again, choose hypoallergenic cleansing products that are suitable for sensitive skin, such as those by Almay or Clinique. The beauty columnist Jemma Kidd (*You Magazine*) recommends using a fragrance-free eye make-up remover such as Liz Earle's Eyebright Soothing Eye Lotion (see Useful Products), which she says doubles up as a desensitising eye compress when applied on a cotton pad. Jemma also recommends Jane Iredale's lavender water-based Dot the i makeup remover swabs to remove eye make up smudges (see Useful Products).

### Do a patch test

If your skin is very sensitive, it's a good idea to do a patch test at least 24 hours before using a new product. Apply a small amount to an inconspicuous area – such as inside your upper arm, or behind an ear.

## Chapter 8

# DIY Complementary Therapies

According to a recent OnePoll survey, 72 per cent of hay fever sufferers prefer to use a natural alternative to conventional medicine, such as acupuncture or homeopathy, to relieve their symptoms. This chapter gives a brief overview and evaluation of complementary therapies that may help to reduce the frequency and severity of hay fever attacks, including acupressure, aromatherapy, homeopathy, reflexology, self-hypnosis and yoga. It includes techniques and treatments you can try for yourself.

The main difference between complementary therapies, often also known as alternative, natural, or holistic therapies, and conventional Western medicine, is that the former approach focuses on treating the individual as a whole, whereas the latter is symptom led. Complementary practitioners view illness as a sign that physical and mental well-being have been disrupted and attempt to restore good health by encouraging the body's own self-healing and self-regulating abilities. They claim that total well-being can be achieved when the mind and body are in a state of balance or 'homeostasis'. Homeostasis is achieved by following the type of lifestyle advocated in this book, i.e. a healthy diet, plenty of fresh air, exercise, sleep and relaxation, combined with stress management and a positive mental attitude.

Unlike drug treatments, which are comparatively recent, complementary therapies such as aromatherapy, massage and reflexology have been used to treat ailments and promote well-being for thousands of years.

## 45. Use aroma power

Essential oils are extracted by various means from the roots, stalks, leaves and flowers of plants.

Aromatherapy is based on the idea that scents released from essential oils affect the hypothalamus, the part of the brain which controls the glands and hormonal system, thus influencing mood and lowering stress levels. As stress is a major hay fever trigger, anything that can relieve stress has the potential to reduce the frequency of attacks. Oils can also relieve symptoms in other ways – some act as decongestants, others are anti-inflammatory, reducing the allergic response. Because essential oils are concentrated, they can sting and cause irritation if applied directly to the skin. Therefore, when used for massage, they should always be diluted in a carrier oil such as olive, sunflower, almond, or wheatgerm before application. Good quality culinary versions will do. The recommended dilution is one or two per cent, depending on the essential oil. One teaspoon of carrier oil contains 100 drops, so add one drop of your chosen essential oil for a one per cent dilution and two drops for a two per cent dilution. Below are some of the essential oils that may help to ease your symptoms.

### First line of attack

Patricia Davis, author of *Aromatherapy An A-Z*, recommends chamomile and melissa oils as her 'first line of attack' to reduce the allergic response that causes hay fever symptoms

Patricia Davis cautions that you should buy oils that are as pure as possible and that you should be suspicious of cheap oils. Reputable suppliers include Tisserand and Baldwins – see Useful Products.

## Chamomile

Try sprinkling a couple of drops of chamomile oil onto a handkerchief and inhale. A massage using a one to two per cent dilution can also be beneficial, as the oil is absorbed into the bloodstream. Many hay fever sufferers claim its soothing, sedative qualities ease their symptoms. There are several types of chamomile – Roman Chamomile and German Chamomile are the most popular. Both have soothing, calming and anti-inflammatory properties. Oil from a type of Mugwort, often sold as Blue Chamomile, should not be used during pregnancy, as it encourages menstruation.

## Melissa (Lemon Balm)

Melissa oil has a soothing, calming effect – both on the mind and body. Patricia Davis says it can sometimes bring about a 'dramatic improvement'. She advises using it in just a one per cent dilution for massage, or sprinkling one or two drops onto a handkerchief.

## Eucalyptus

A steam inhalation of eucalptus oil is especially helpful for a stuffy nose and sinusitis, as it has decongestant and expectorant properties. Alternatively, sprinkle two or three drops onto a handkerchief.

### Steam inhalation

Add three or four drops of your chosen essential oil to a bowl of boiling water. Once the water has cooled slightly, drape a towel over your face and head and inhale the vapours. Caution: inhale the steam for just 30 seconds the first time. If there is no adverse reaction, gradually increase the inhalation time to three to five minutes.

## Lavender

A steam inhalation containing lavender oil can help to ease sneezing and a runny nose. Lavender can also relieve stress, which is often both a cause and effect of hay fever. Having a stuffy nose can disrupt sleep – sprinkle just two or three drops of lavender oil on your pillow to help you drop off. Don't use lavender oil in the first three months of pregnancy. Don't use at all if there is a history of miscarriage.

## Peppermint

Peppermint oil helps to relieve nasal congestion, sinusitis pain and headache. The active ingredient, menthol, is often a component of products designed to deal with these symptoms. For a blocked nose, sprinkle two to three drops of oil on a handkerchief and inhale. For sinusitis, use it in a steam inhalation. To relieve both sinusitis pain and headache, make a compress by soaking a clean cotton handkerchief or facecloth in a bowl of lukewarm water containing four drops of peppermint oil. Wring out any excess moisture and apply to the affected areas. Peppermint is a stimulant, so don't use it close to bedtime. It shouldn't be used during pregnancy.

### Rose

Rose oil has an uplifting fragrance and anti-depressant properties, making it especially useful when your hay fever symptoms are getting you down. Try adding a few drops to a warm bath, or enjoy a massage with this aromatic oil, using a one to two per cent dilution. Avoid rose oil in the first three months of pregnancy. Don't use at all if there is a history of miscarriage.

### Bergamot

Bergamot oil is also uplifting and relaxing, helping to relieve depression, tension and anxiety. Use it for massage or add it to the bath, diluted in a carrier oil, when your hay fever symptoms are making you feel low. Use bergamot in no more than a one per cent dilution – in higher strengths it can increase the skin's sensitivity to sunlight, making it more likely to burn.

### Rosemary

Rosemary oil is excellent for the respiratory problems experienced with hay fever. It acts as a decongestant and is renowned for its ability to 'clear the head'. Try using it in a steam inhalation, or put one or two drops on a handkerchief. Don't use rosemary oil during pregnancy, or if you suffer from epilepsy.

## 46. Help yourself with homeopathy

Homeopathy aims to treat the whole person by taking not just physical symptoms into account, but also character and emotions.

It's thought that the Greek physician Hippocrates initiated homeopathy when he introduced the idea that 'like cures like'; substances that in large doses cause symptoms in a well person can relieve the same symptoms, in small doses, in an ill person. Homeopathy literally means 'same suffering'.

In the sixteenth century, a Swiss doctor called Paracelsus developed the concept, suggesting that plants and metals contained ingredients that could help the body to self-heal. In the late eighteenth century, a doctor called Samuel Hahnemann began testing substances such as quinine, arsenic and belladonna on himself and family members, and noted the results. He produced a book outlining his findings and began treating patients with his remedies, which he produced by diluting small doses of substances. He called his new treatment system 'homeopathy'. Although the medical establishment dismissed Hahnemann's theories, homeopathy flourished during the nineteenth century. However, by the early twentieth century, there were differences in opinion as to how homeopathy should be practised. Some believed a person's emotional characteristics should be taken into account and high potencies used, whilst others favoured prescribing according to physical symptoms, using lower doses. This disagreement weakened homepathy's position against conventional medicine. However, since the late twentieth century, homeopathy has enjoyed a revival as people have become disenchanted with the side effects of conventional drugs.

In homeopathy, symptoms such as inflammation or fever are seen as a sign that the body is attempting to heal itself. Homeopathic remedies are designed to stimulate this self-healing process and this will often lead to a temporary worsening of symptoms before the condition improves.

The substances used in homeopathic remedies are derived from plant, animal and mineral sources. These are crushed and turned into a tincture that is then diluted many times. Homeopaths claim that the more diluted a remedy is, the higher its potency and the lower its potential side effects. This idea is based on the 'memory of water' theory, which claims that, although molecules from substances are diluted until it is unlikely that any remain, they leave behind an electromagnetic 'footprint' – like a recording on an audiotape – which exerts an effect on the body.

These ideas are controversial, with many in the medical profession remaining sceptical. However, in 2003, a review of research into the use of homeopathy concluded that it had a 'positive treatment effect' in eight health conditions – one of which was hay fever.

There are two main types of remedy – whole person based and symptom based. A homeopath would prescribe a remedy based on your personality, as well as the symptoms you experience. However, the easiest way to treat yourself is to select the remedy that most closely matches your individual symptoms. Below are some of the homeopathic remedies commonly prescribed for hay fever and the symptoms for which they're indicated. You can buy homeopathic remedies in most pharmacies and health food shops. Alternatively, visit www.healthroughhomeopathy.com, a website that offers information about homeopathy and useful resources, including an interactive hay fever questionnaire that enables you to select the correct remedy for your particular symptoms. You could also try Helios Homeopathy, a homeopathic pharmacy with an online shop (see Directory).

### Not a quick fix

Practitioners caution people that homeopathy isn't a 'quick fix' – the remedies may take a while to take effect. Homeopathic remedies are generally considered safe and don't have any known side effects, although sometimes a temporary worsening of symptoms, known as 'aggravation' may take place. This is seen as a good sign, as it suggests that the remedy is encouraging the healing process. If this happens, stop taking the remedy and wait for your symptoms to improve. If there is steady improvement, don't restart the remedy. If the improvement stops, resume taking the remedy.

### Allium cepa

A remedy derived from onions that is suggested for a streaming nose with a reddened and inflamed nostril and upper lip area, often accompanied by a headache and sore throat. The symptoms are worse in warm rooms and improved by fresh air.

### Arsenic iodide

For hay fever with a constant need to sneeze, honey-coloured catarrh, sore nostrils, a burning throat and an irritating cough. Symptoms are made worse by sneezing, warmth and dry weather and improved by rest, eating and fresh air.

## Euphrasia officinalis

This remedy is derived from the herb eyebright, which has traditonally been used to treat eye conditions. It is used where the eyes are badly affected with inflammation, itching and watering. The eyelids may also be swollen and inflamed. There may be a clear discharge from the nose, a cough and a sore throat. These symptoms improve with lying down in a darkened room and are exacerbated by warm, windy weather and bright light.

## Galphimia glauca

Galphimia glauca (golden thryallis) is particularly recommended for sore and itchy eyes, and has been used for the treatment of asthma and allergies in Latin American traditional medicine. A review of seven different placebo-controlled trials concluded that a homeopathic remedy derived from this plant was beneficial in 79 per cent of 752 hay fever cases, relieving eye and nose symptoms as effectively as conventional antihistamine medications.

## Mixed pollens

This is a remedy made from various hay fever triggers including flower, grass and tree pollens, which means that, strictly speaking, it is an isopathic remedy as it uses the cause of the symptoms, rather than treating like with like. A Scottish study in *The Lancet* in 1986, and a controlled clinical trial in Phoenix, Arizona in 2005, suggested that this type of homeopathic remedy could help to reduce symptoms.

## Sabadilla officinale

Recommended when the main symptom is a sore throat that is relieved by warm food and drinks. The eyes may water, especially outdoors, and the eyelids are inflamed and red. The nose is very itchy and there is repeated sneezing, and the insides of the ears may also feel itchy. Sabadilla is often combined with Allium cepa and Euphrasia officinalis to make hay fever remedies, such as Nelsons Pollenna (see Useful Products).

## Solanum dulcamara

This is a remedy made from the stems and leaves of *Solanum dulcamara*, also known as bittersweet and woody nightshade, a plant with anti-inflammatory properties. Recommended for nasal congestion, constricted breathing and watery eyes, especially where grass pollen, dust mites and other allergens increase symptoms. Symptoms are exacerbated by cold damp weather and worse at night, and they are improved with warmth and physical activity.

## Wyethia

Recommended for an itchy nose, ears, palate and throat, accompanied by violent sneezing but very little nasal discharge and a dry and swollen throat. Symptoms are worse after physical activity and eating.

## Combination H tissue salts

Though not strictly a homeopathic remedy, tissue salts are prepared homeopathically from minerals such as quartz and rock salt. Dr William Schussler, a homeopathic doctor who believed that mineral deficiencies left the body weakened and more susceptible to disease, devised these remedies in the 1870s. Combination H, recommended for the relief of hay fever and allergic rhinitis, contains Mag. Phos. (Magnesium Phosphate), Nat. Mur. (Sodium Chloride) and Silica (Silicon Dioxide). (The details of this item are listed under 'New Era Combination H Tissue Salts' in Useful Products.)

## 47. Apply acupressure

Acupressure is part of traditional Chinese medicine and is often referred to as 'acupuncture without needles', as it works on the same points on the body. Like acupuncture, it's based on the idea that life energy, or *qi*, flows through channels in the body known as meridians. An even passage of *qi* throughout the body is viewed as necessary to good health. Disruption of the flow of *qi* in a meridian can lead to illness at any point along it. The flow of *qi* can be affected by various lifestyle factors, including stress, emotional distress, diet and environment.

*Qi* is most concentrated at points along the meridians known as acupoints. Using the fingers and thumbs to apply firm but gentle pressure to these points stimulates the body's natural self-healing abilities. Muscular tension is relieved and the circulation boosted, thereby promoting good health. The application of pressure also seems to stimulate the production of endorphins – the body's natural painkillers.

Whilst there doesn't appear to have been any research into the effectiveness of acupressure for the relief of hay fever symptoms, there have been a number of studies which suggest that acupuncture may be beneficial. An Australian study in 2007 involving 80 hay fever sufferers concluded that acupuncture reduced symptoms and the need for medication. Another controlled trial in Germany in 2008 reported that treating hay fever sufferers with acupuncture alongside routine treatments improved their symptoms. Many Chinese people use acupressure to self-treat a range of common conditions.

## Wind pool

These two acupoints, also known as *Fengchi*, were used in the Australian study mentioned above. They can be found at the base of the skull on either side of the neck bone. Applying firm pressure with the index and middle fingers for up to two minutes is thought to relieve congestion in the sinuses.

## Bend pool

This is also known as the *Quchi* acupoint. Fold your right arm across your chest, then use your left thumb to apply firm pressure to the outer edge of the crease on the inside of your right elbow joint. Repeat on the left arm, using the right thumb. Applying pressure to this acupoint is believed to ease itchy eyes and clear blocked sinuses. You can also buy an acupressure band that applies constant pressure to this acupoint. See the Hay-Band in the Useful Products section for more details.

## Welcome fragrance

These are also known as the *Yingxiang* acupoints, which were among those used in the Australian study. These two acupoints can be located at the lower outer edge of each nostril. Applying firm pressure with each index finger for up to two minutes is thought to relieve sinus pain.

## Seal hall

This acupoint, also known as *Yintang*, which is situated between the eyebrows, was also used in the Australian study. Using both index fingers to apply firm pressure to this area for up to two minutes is claimed to ease a runny nose.

## 48. Relax with reflexology

Reflexology is based on the theory that points on the feet, hands and face, known as reflexes, correspond to parts of the body, glands and organs. Stimulating these reflexes using the fingers and thumbs is thought to bring about physiological changes, which encourage the mind and body to self-heal. Practitioners claim that imbalances in the body result in granular deposits in the relevant reflex, leading to tenderness. Corns, bunions and even hard skin are believed to indicate problems in the parts of the body to which their position is linked. Whilst medical opinion is divided, evidence suggests that foot and hand massage can reduce stress.

### Simple hand reflexology

Use your right thumb to apply pressure to your left palm, starting just above the wrist and working from left to right. Continue working across the palm from left to right until you reach the base of the fingers. Repeat on your right palm, using your left thumb. Ann Gillanders, a reflexologist and author of *A Gaia Busy Person's Guide to Reflexology*, recommends applying pressure to the entire palm area of each hand to stimulate the digestive and respiratory system reflexes and to help relieve allergy symptoms.

## 49. Try self-hypnosis

Trance-like states have been used for centuries by different cultures to encourage healing. The founder of modern hypnosis was Franz

Anton Mesmer, whose method of treating patients was termed 'mesmerism'. Hypnotherapists promote a state of mind that's similar to daydreaming and encourages deep relaxation and openness to suggestion.

Studies suggest that as well as being relaxing – which in itself can be beneficial to hay fever sufferers – self-hypnosis may boost immune function and reduce symptoms. A two-year study in Switzerland in 2005 concluded that self-hypnosis may help hay fever sufferers. Participants with moderate to severe hay fever received between two and five lessons in self-hypnosis. They then practised the techniques over two hay fever seasons and recorded their symptoms. This group showed a marked improvement in symptoms like a runny nose and needed fewer doses of medication, compared to the control group, who did not learn self-hypnosis. In the second year, the control group also learned self-hypnosis and displayed the same improvements as the first group.

## Simple self-hypnosis

Most people can learn safe and simple self-hypnosis techniques. The following steps will take you through a basic self-hypnosis, which could aid relaxation and positive thinking and possibly help to ease hay fever symptoms.

1. Lie or sit comfortably in a quiet place, where you're unlikely to be disturbed.

2. Focus on your breathing – breathe slowly and deeply.

3. Start counting backwards from 300. If your mind starts to drift away, simply start counting backwards again.

4. At the same time, start relaxing each part of your body. Allow the muscles in your face to relax, then those in your neck and shoulders, back, arms, legs and finally your feet.

5. Now repeat affirmations – positive statements about yourself – as though they're already true, e.g. 'I can breathe easily and feel great when I am outdoors.'

6. As you make your affirmation, experience it in your subconscious, as though it's happening now, by visualising a scene in which you've already achieved your goal.

7. It is claimed that the more senses you use in your visualisation, the more effective it is likely to be. For example, picture yourself walking in a beautiful park full of flowers. Imagine breathing in the fresh air, smelling the flowers' fragrance and feeling really well.

8. When you're ready to come out of your trance, start counting to ten, telling yourself 'When I reach five I'll start to awaken; when I reach ten I'll wake up, feeling calm and relaxed.'

## 50. Breathe more easily with yoga

Practising yoga may help to ease your symptoms by reducing stress levels, which are often both a cause and effect of hay fever. Also, certain *asanas* (postures) and breathing exercises may expand the chest area and improve breathing. The word 'yoga' comes from the Sanskrit word *Yuj*, meaning union. Yoga postures and breathing exercises are aimed at uniting the mind, body and soul. Below are some of the breathing exercises (*pranyama*) and *asanas* that may help ease your symptoms when practised regularly.

## Cleansing breath (*Kapalabhati*)

This breathing technique expels air and waste from the respiratory passages and is believed to help ease sinus problems caused by excess mucus.

1. Sit comfortably with your spine straight.

2. Inhale deeply, allowing your tummy to inflate.

3. Exhale rapidly and forcefully as you pull in your tummy muscles.

4. Relax and passively allow the next inhalation to happen.

5. Repeat up to 20 times to a steady rhythm.

## Alternate nostril breathing (*Nadi Shodana*)

This breathing exercise helps to clear the nasal passages and promotes calm.

1. Place the index and middle fingers of your right hand in between your eyebrows.

2. Press your right nostril closed with your thumb. Inhale slowly through left nostril.

3. Holding your breath, release your right nostril and block your left nostril with your ring finger.

4. Exhale slowly through your right nostril. Then release the left nostril and inhale.

5. Repeat this cycle five to ten times.

## The cobra (*Bhujangasana*)

The cobra may be helpful to hay fever sufferers because it promotes deep breathing and improves chest expansion.

1. Lie face down on the floor with your legs and feet together.

2. Place your hands on each side of your chest, fingers apart and pointing forwards, in line with your shoulders.

3. Inhale, straightening your elbows and lifting your chest. Arch your spine and roll back your shoulders.

4. Slowly return to your original position, exhaling.

5. Roll onto your back and hug your knees into your chest.

## The bow (*Dhanurasana*)

The bow posture expands the chest, helping to strengthen the respiratory system.

1. Lie on your tummy with your arms at your sides and your palms facing upwards.

2. Bend your knees and bring your heels towards your bottom.

3. Reach backwards and grasp your ankles, resting your weight on your tummy.

4. Lift your knees higher by pulling your ankles, lifting your chest and arching your back.

5. Roll onto your back and hug your knees close to your chest.

## Learn yoga

The best and probably the most fun way to learn yoga is to attend classes run by a qualified teacher. To find one near you, go to the

British Wheel of Yoga's website – www.bwy.org.uk. If you'd prefer to teach yourself at home, visit www.abc-of-yoga.com, a site which shows you how to do the various postures using animated clips. You can also buy CD and MP3 hatha yoga class downloads, suitable for all levels and abilities and download a free 'taster session' at www.yoga2hear.co.uk. You can also find yoga information, products and guidance at www.yoga-abode.com.

## Safe yoga

When practising yoga at home, always proceed gently and avoid forcing your body into the postures. Always stop if you feel any discomfort. Wear lightweight, loose clothing, to allow you to move freely and no footwear, as yoga is best performed barefoot. Use a non-slip mat if the floor is slippery. Don't attempt inverted postures if you have a neck or back problem or have high blood pressure or heart or circulatory problems. If in doubt, consult your GP first.

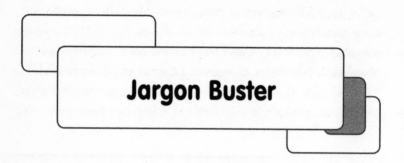

**Jargon Buster**

Listed below are the meanings of terms that may be used in connection with hay fever.

**Allergen** – any substance, pollen, dust, etc., that causes an allergic reaction.

**Allergy** – an extreme response by the immune system to a normally harmless substance, involving the production of a harmful antibody known as IgE.

**Anaphylaxis** – also known as anaphylactic shock. A severe and potentially fatal allergic reaction.

**Antihistamine** – a drug that blocks the effects of histamine.

**Anti-inflammatory** – a drug or other substance that counteracts inflammation.

**Atopic** – allergic.

**Chronic** – persistent, long-lasting.

**Decongestant** – A type of medicine that reduces swelling (congestion) in the nose and the chest and can clear a stuffy nose, making it easier to breathe.

**Double-blind** – a trial in which information that may influence the behaviour of the investigators or the participants (such as if participants have been given a placebo rather than an active treatment) is withheld.

**Histamine** – a substance released by the immune system in response to an allergy.

**Immunoglobulin E** – a harmful antibody usually known as IgE.

**Inflammation** – a response by the immune system designed to protect the body from invasion by foreign substances or infections. The effects can include increased mucus production, swelling, redness, heat and pain.

**Mould** – a type of fungus that can cause allergic reactions when the tiny spores they give off are inhaled.

**Mucous membrane** – membrane in the body that produces mucus, such as that found in the nasal passages, mouth and throat.

**Mucus** – a sticky substance produced in different parts of the body, including the nasal passages, airways and sinuses.

**Pollen** – fine, powdery grains produced by flowering plants, grasses, trees and weeds to produce new plants.

**Prostaglandins** – hormone-like substances made in the body from essential fatty acids, some of which promote inflammation, whilst others reduce it.

**Sensitivity** – a response by the immune system to a particular substance.

**Steroids (corticosteroids)** – drugs with anti-inflammatory properties, similar to the steroid hormones produced by the adrenal glands.

# Helpful Reading

Black, Octavius and Bailey, Sebastian, *The Mind Gym: Give Me Time* (Time Warner Books, 2006). This book shows you how to reduce stress and use your time wisely by striking a balance between work and play and doing things that engage you and give you a sense of purpose.

Carlson, Richard, *Don't Sweat the Small Stuff... and it's all Small Stuff: Simple Ways to Keep the Little Things from Taking Over Your Life* (Mobius, 1998). This book offers some effective strategies to help you achieve inner calm.

Davis, Patricia, *Aromatherapy – An A-Z* (Vermillion, 2005). A comprehensive guide to essential oils and how to use them to reduce stress and improve your health.

Gillanders, Ann, *A Gaia Busy Person's Guide to Reflexology* (Gaia Books Ltd, 2006). An indispensable self-help guide to reflexology.

Hoffman, David, *The Herbal Handbook: A User's Guide to Medical Herbalism* (Inner Traditions Bear and Company, 1998). An excellent guide to a wide range of medicinal herbs, including their uses and their effects on the body.

Jarvis, Deforest Clinton, *Folk Medicine: A famous doctor's guide to folk medicine practices of Vermont – the nature secrets of honey, apple cider vinegar and foods for good health* (Fawcett Books, 1995). This book was first published in 1958 and contains the natural health secrets of people living in Vermont in the US.

Savill, Antoinette, *Gluten, Wheat and Dairy Free Cookbook: Over 200 Allergy-free Recipes from the Sensitive Gourmet* (Thorsons, 2000). A useful cookery book for hay fever sufferers who have linked their symptoms to food allergies.

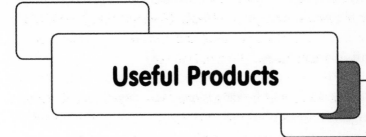

# Useful Products

Below is a list of products that may help to prevent or relieve hay fever symptoms. The author doesn't endorse or recommend any particular product and this list is by no means exhaustive – there is a vast range of products that may help.

### 4-in-1 Display Digital Thermo-Hygrometer and Clock
A compact thermo-hygrometer that measures humidity and temperature as well as displaying the time. It can be free standing or wall mounted and is suitable for use in the home.
Website: www.humidifiers-shop.co.uk

### Air Tamer Ionic Air Purifier for the Car
An air purifier that plugs into a cigarette lighter and clears allergens, such as pollen, dust and fuel fumes.
Website: www.allergybestbuys.co.uk

### AllerGForte
A supplement containing stinging nettle extract, vitamin C, quercetin, ginger powder and turmeric that claims to maintain a healthy immune system. Available from health food stores.
Website: www.healthaid.co.uk

### Allerpet

A dry shampoo that removes allergens from pets' skin and fur.
Website: www.demite.com/allerpet/

### Anti-Allergen Spray

A spray containing natural ingredients that can be safely applied to upholstery, animal bedding, clothes and carpets, etc. to reduce allergens for up to 30 days.
Website: www.allergymatters.com

### Baldwins Butterbur

Available in root, tablet or capsule form.
Website: www.baldwins.co.uk

### Baldwins Elderberry Herbal Tincture

A herbal tincture containing elderberries that can be added to water or fruit juice.
Website: www.baldwins.co.uk

### Baldwins Elderflower Herbal Tincture

A herbal tincture containing elderflower that can be added to water or fruit juice.
Website: www.baldwins.co.uk

### Baldwins Essential Oils

A comprehensive range of good quality essential oils.
Website: www.baldwins.co.uk

### Breathe Right Nasal Strips

Self-adhesive strips that attach to the outside of the nose to help keep the nasal passages open during sleep. By dilating the nasal passage, Breathe Right Nasal Strips can provide temporary relief from sinus congestion. May be used during sleep or during the day.
Website: www.boots.com

### Clipper Organic Nettle Tea

Tea made from organically grown young nettle leaves.
Website: www.goodnessdirect.co.uk

### Dot the i makeup remover swabs

Jane Iredale's lavender water-based make-up remover swabs calm and condition the skin around the eye area and are ideal for removing eye make-up smudges.
Website: www.jiproducts.co.uk

### Ecover

A range of ecological, petrochemical-free products, including household cleaners, laundry liquids and powders and washing-up liquids, that are based on plant and mineral ingredients.
Website: www.ecover.com

### Glucasan

Contains beta-glucans from baker's yeast, which are thought to normalise immune function and help reduce allergies.
Website: www.vitalizehealth.co.uk

### Guduchi (*Tinospora cordifolia*)

Capsules containing guduchi (*Tinospora cordifolia*), a herb used in Ayurvedic medicine to boost the immune system.
Website: www.buyayurvedic.com

### Hambleden Organic Elderflower Teabags

Teabags containing organic elderflowers.

Website: www.greenlife.co.uk

### Hay-Band

A latex-free acupressure band that fits around the arm at the elbow. It has a plastic stud which applies pressure and stimulates the *QuiChi* pressure point.

Website: www.healthy-house.co.uk

### HayMax

HayMax is a balm that works as an effective pollen barrier when applied to the bottom of the nose. It contains organic beeswax, seed oil and essential oils. There are four varieties: Aloe Vera, Lavender, Pure, or Frankincense.

Website: www.haybalm.f2s.com

### Heaven Fresh Car Air Purifier XJ-600

Ionic air purifier that plugs into your cigarette lighter socket. Removes pollen, mould spores, cigarette smoke and dust from the air inside your car.

Website: www.boots.com

### HEPA Air Purifier

HEPA stands for High Efficiency Particulate Arresting. HEPA filters contain several layers of fibre that trap up to 99 per cent of tiny airborne particles, including pollen, dust mites and dust.

Website: www.hepaairpurifiers.co.uk

## Ion Life Car Air Filter & Ioniser

In-car air filter with a five-stage filtration system that traps pollen, dust, etc. and eliminates cigarette smoke and fungal spores.
Website: www.energiseyourlife.com

## Iredale Mineral Make-Up

Recommended by Sheherazade Goldsmith, editor of the book *A Slice of Organic Life*, who uses these products on her sensitive skin. The range includes foundations, powders, lipsticks and glosses, eyeshadows, eyeliners and mascara.
Website: www.jiproducts.co.uk

## Lily Lolo Mineral Cosmetics

This range includes foundations, powders, blushers, bronzers and eyeshadows. All products are paraben and fragrance free.
Website: www.lilylolo.co.uk

## Liz Earle's Eyebright Soothing Eye Lotion

Gentle eye lotion containing the herb eyebright, witch hazel, organic aloe vera and cornflower to cool and refresh puffy, irritated eyes.
Website: www.lizearle.com

## Luffa Complex

Contains sponge cucumber (*Luffa operculata*), golden thryallis (*Galphimia glauca*), and other herb extracts to relieve hay fever symptoms. Available as a tincture, tablets and nasal spray. The nasal spray eases a blocked, runny or itchy nose.
Website: www.avogel.co.uk

## MediBee's Famous Pollen Capsules

A pollen supplement. Taking pollen orally is believed to lower the body's sensitivity to it.

Website: www.allergybestbuys.co.uk

## Medinose

A hand-held device, suitable for all ages, that uses phototherapy to reduce hay fever symptoms. It consists of a small power pack and two probes, which are inserted into the nostrils. Recommended use is four-and-a-half minutes, two to three times a day. Suitable for all ages.

Website: www.anhealth.co.uk

## MicroAirScreen re-usable Face Mask

A reusable mask for use indoors or outdoors to protect against inhaled allergens such as dust, pollen and pet allergens. Ideal for use when gardening and mowing the lawn.

Website: www.allergybestbuys.co.uk

## Multibionta

A multivitamin and mineral supplement containing three probiotics – one strain of *Lactobacillus* and two of *Bifidobacterium*. The tablets are enteric coated to prevent stomach acids from destroying the probiotics. There are five different reasonably priced formulas to suit different age groups and lifestyles.

Website: www.multibionta.co.uk

## NasalAir Guard

A nose filter made from clear, medical-grade plastic that fits discreetly across the nostrils and prevents pollen and other substances from being inhaled.

Website: www.nasalairguard.com

## Nelsons Pollenna

Nelsons Pollenna contains the remedies Allium cepa, Euphrasia officinalis and Sabadilla officinarum, which homeopaths commonly use to treat hay fever.

Website: www.nelsonshomeopathy.co.uk

## New Era Combination H tissue salts

A homoeopathically prepared biochemic remedy for hay fever and allergic rhinitis.

Website: www.seven-seas.com

## PetalCleanse

A surfactant-based lotion that safely removes allergens from the coats of cats and dogs. It has been independently tested and found to be effective in reducing symptoms in over 90 per cent of people who are allergic to pets.

Website: www.healthy-house.co.uk

## Potters Allerclear

A range of herbal products for the relief of hay fever symptoms. The nasal spray contains dead sea salt to relieve congestion and irritation, the eye drops contain eyebright to ease irritation and dryness, and the tablets contain garlic and echinacea to reduce catarrh and congestion.

Website: www.herbal-direct.com

## Puravent Car Pollen Filter

A pollen filter that you can fit yourself. It is available in various sizes to fit popular makes and models of car.

Website: www.puravent.co.uk

### Pycnogenol Pine Bark Extract

Tablets containing pycnogenol, which is believed to relieve hay fever symptoms.

Website: www.healthydirect.co.uk

### Salitair Salt Therapy Salt Pipe

A pipe containing salt crystals which, when inhaled, cleanse the respiratory tract and encourage self-cleansing mechanisms. It claims to thin mucus and ease breathing.

Website:www.healthandcare.co.uk

### Sambucol Black Elderberry Liquid Extract Immuno Forte Formula

A sugar-free elderberry liquid extract that contains natural antioxidants and added vitamin C, zinc and propolis and which may help maintain healthy immune function. Not recommended for children under 12 or pregnant women.

Website: www.boots.com

### Sterimar Sea Water Nasal Spray

Anti-inflammatory nasal spray based on sea water. Clears mucus from the nose, easing congestion.

Website: www.boots.com

### Tisserand Aromatherapy Pure Essential Oils

A wide range of good-quality essential oils designed to improve health and happiness.

Website: www.tisserand.com

### Weleda Mixed Pollen Tablets

Homeopathic remedy containing mixed pollens.

Website: www.weleda.co.uk

## Window-filta

A removable electrostatic air filter for windows that is designed to enable hay fever and asthma sufferers to sleep with their windows open. The filter fits to your open window, allowing a free passage of air but trapping pollen, spore, diesel particles and dust.

Website: www.allergybestbuys.co.uk

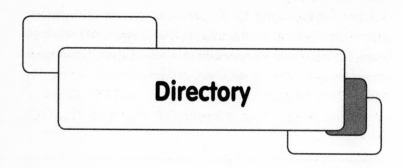

# Directory

Below is a list of contacts offering products, information and support for hay fever sufferers.

## ABC of Yoga

A website offering tips, advice and poses for those who wish to practise yoga at home. Also provides meditation techniques.
Website: www.abc-of-yoga.com

## Action Against Allergy

A UK charity that aims to advance understanding and recognition of allergic medical conditions and allergy-related illness. Members can access information about allergies and doctors and clinics that specialise in their treatment. There is also a newsletter and a telephone network that enables members to talk to fellow allergy sufferers.
Address: Action Against Allergy, PO Box 278, Twickenham TW1 4QQ
Telephone: 0208 89 22 711
Email: AAA@actionagainstallergy.freeserve.co.uk
Website: www.actionagainstallergy.co.uk

## The AAIR Charity

A charity that raises funds for the asthma, allergy and inflammation research unit based at Southampton General Hospital. The research team aims to find effective treatments for allergic diseases. The website offers information about allergies, including hay fever and asthma.

Address: The AAIR Charity, AIR, Mailpoint 810, Level F, Southampton General Hospital, Tremona Road, Southampton, Hampshire, SO16 6YD

Telephone: 02380 771 234

Email: caroline@aaircharity.org

Website: www.aaircharity.org

## Allergymatters

A website selling a huge range of products to help combat allergies, including air purifiers and natural cleaners and remedies.

Telephone: 0208 33 90 029

Website: www.allergymatters.com

## Allergy Answers

Website endorsed by Allergy UK that provides useful information about hay fever and other allergies.

www.allergyanswers.co.uk

## Allergy UK (formerly The British Allergy Foundation)

A nationwide medical charity for people with allergies, food intolerances and chemical sensitivities. Provides up-to-date information on all aspects of allergies, as well as a nationwide network of support contacts offering advice and support to fellow sufferers, online forums and an e-newsletter. It also runs three product endorsement schemes to help allergy sufferers select 'allergy friendly' products, such as air purifiers, as well as listing alerts on allergens in particular products.

Address: Allergy UK, 3 White Oak Square, London Road, Swanley, Kent, BR8 7AG
Telephone: 01322 619 898
Email: info@allergyuk.org
Website: www.allergyuk.org

## Asthma UK

A UK charity aimed at improving the health and well-being of asthma sufferers. As well as funding research into the condition, it publishes reports and offers a magazine, newsletter and helpline. As hay fever is often linked to asthma, it provides useful information for hay fever sufferers too.
Address: Asthma UK, Summit House, 70 Wilson Street, London, EC2A 2DB
Telephone: 0207 78 64 900
Email: info@asthma.org.uk
Website: www.asthma.org.uk

## Blossom

A children's campaign from Allergy UK that aims to provide support to child allergy sufferers and their families.
Address: Blossom Campaign, Allergy UK, 3 White Oak Square, London Road, Swanley, Kent, BR8 7AG
Telephone: 01322 619 898
Website: www.blossomcampaign.org

## British Society for Allergy and Clinical Immunology

Professional society of allergists and clinical immunologists. Lists specialist NHS Allergy Clinics and Clinical Immunologists in the UK.
Address: Elliott House, 10–12 Allington Street, London, SW1E 5EH
Telephone: 0207 80 87 135
Website: www.bsaci.org

## Hayfever Expert

A website that aims to offer a unique reference point on coping with and relieving hay fever.

Website: www.hayfeverexpert.co.uk

## Health Boards

Health Boards provide message boards on various conditions, including allergies.

Website: www.healthboards.com

## Helios Homeopathy

A homeopathic pharmacy with an online shop. Offers over 3,000 homeopathic remedies.

Address: Helios Homoeopathy Ltd, 89–97 Camden Rd, Tunbridge Wells, Kent, TN1 2QR

Telephone: 01892 537 254

Website: www.helios.co.uk

## HouseDustMite.org

A website offering detailed information about the house dust mite and how it can be linked to allergic rhinitis and asthma. Includes advice on how to control house dust mites.

Website: www.housedustmite.org

## Kids' Allergies

Website set up to offer information about the causes and treatments of allergies in children.

Website: www.kidsallergies.co.uk

## Medicines and Healthcare products Regulatory Agency (MHRA)

A government agency responsible for ensuring that medicines and medical devices work and are acceptably safe.
Address: 10–2 Market Towers, 1 Nine Elms Lane, London, SW8 5NQ
Telephone: 0207 084 2000 / 0207 210 3000
Email: info@mhra.gsi.gov.uk
Website: www.mhra.gov.uk

## Midlands Asthma and Allergy Research Association (MAARA)

MAARA is a registered charity based in the East Midlands that was founded in 1968 by Dr Harry Morrow Brown to undertake and fund research into the causes of asthma and allergies. It also aims to raise the profile of allergic conditons and provides useful information, including pollen and spore updates for hay fever and asthma sufferers in the East Midlands.
Address: PO Box 1057, Leicester, LE2 3GZ
Telephone: 01332 799 600
Email: enquiries@maara.org
Website: www.maara.org

## National Pollen and Aerobiology Research Unit (NPARU)

NPARU is the only pollen forecast organisation that has access to data from the UK pollen and spore monitoring network. It has 20 sites as far north as Invergowrie in north-east Scotland and as far south as the Isle of Wight, which are run by various institutions, including universities and colleges, hospital allergy clinics and environmental health offices. It offers information on pollen, including a pollen calendar, which shows when the main allergenic plants are in flower.
Website: http://pollenuk.worc.ac.uk

## Netweather

Netweather is an independent weather forecasting company. The company's website provides detailed weather and pollen forecasts.
Website: www.netweather.tv

## Pollenforecast.org

A link to the pollen and fungal spore forecasts and calendars on the Zirtek Allergy website, which are based on data provided by the National Pollen and Aerobiology Research Unit (NPARU).
Website: www.pollenforecast.org

## Relaxation for Living Institute

A charity that offers information on stress and its effects on the body, as well as relaxation techniques. It also provides a database of Relaxation for Living Institute teachers and relaxation classes across the UK.
Address: Relaxation for Living Institute, 1 Great Chapel Street, London, W1F 8FA
Telephone: 0207 439 4277 or 0207 437 5880
Website: www.rfli.co.uk

## The Soap Kitchen

A company that sells a range of ingredients, such as borax, bicarbonate of soda and essential oils, from which you can make your own cleaning products.
Address: Units 2 D&E Hatchmoor Industrial Estate, Hatchmoor Road, Torrington, Devon, EX38 7HP
Telephone: 01805 622 944
Email: info@thesoapkitchen.co.uk
Website: www.thesoapkitchen.co.uk

### The Stress Management Society
A society formed in 2003 by healthcare professionals and recognised as a leading authority on stress management issues. Its website offers advice on dealing with stress, a free stress guide and a monthly e-newsletter.
Telephone: 0844 357 8629
Email: info@stress.org.uk
Website: www.stress.org.uk

### Talk Allergy
Website offering information, a message board, an e-newsletter and a pen pal area for allergy sufferers.
Website: www.talkallergy.com

### UK Air Quality Archive
A government website that provides regional air pollution forecasts and bulletins for the UK, as well as general information about pollution and its effects on health.
Freephone: 0800 55 66 77
Email: aqinfo@aeat.co.uk
Website: www.airquality.co.uk

# Other titles in the Personal Health Guides series include:

*50 Things You Can Do Today to Manage Eczema*
*50 Things You Can Do Today to Manage IBS*
*50 Things You Can Do Today to Manage Insomnia*
*50 Things You Can Do Today to Manage Menopause*
*50 Things You Can Do Today to Manage Migraines*

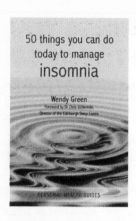

50 things you can do today to manage insomnia

Wendy Green

Foreword by Dr Chris Idzikowski
Director of the Edinburgh Sleep Centre

PERSONAL HEALTH GUIDES

# 50 THINGS YOU CAN DO TODAY TO MANAGE INSOMNIA

Wendy Green

ISBN: 978 1 84024 723 7

Paperback £5.99

Do you lie awake in bed worrying about things
you have to do the next day?

Do you get up feeling tired and as if
you haven't had enough sleep?

If so, you could be suffering from insomnia. In this easy-to-follow book, Wendy Green explains the sleep/wake cycle, and offers practical advice and a holistic approach to help you combat insomnia, including simple lifestyle and dietary changes and DIY complementary therapies.

'… *this book helpfully provides a comprehensive rundown of everything that might impact on sleep and help the insomniac... All in all a fun read in which even the most committed insomniac will find solace*'

Dr Chris Idzikowski, director of the Edinburgh Sleep Centre

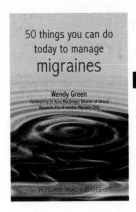

# 50 THINGS YOU CAN DO TODAY TO MANAGE MIGRAINES

Wendy Green

ISBN: 978 1 84024 722 0

Paperback     £5.99

Do you suffer from severe headaches, sometimes with nausea and visual impairment?

Can these headaches last for up to a day or longer at a time?

If so, you could be experiencing migraines. In this easy-to-follow book, Wendy Green explains how dietary, psychological and environmental factors can cause migraines, and offers practical advice and a holistic approach to help you manage them, including simple lifestyle and dietary changes and DIY complementary therapies.

'Wendy Green outlines the variety of treatments that are available over the counter, and also gives an overview of what is available from a GP… It may not yet be possible to 'cure' migraines but it is possible to lead a normal life despite them'

Dr Anne MacGregor, director of clinical research,
City of London Migraine Clinic

Have you enjoyed this book?
If so, why not write a review on your favourite website?

Thanks very much for buying this Summersdale book.

www.summersdale.com